MW01598314

EMPIRE Publishing
20212 Champion Forest Dr. #303
Spring, TX 77379
www.empireghostwriter.com/book-process
@empirepubishing

Legal & Disclaimer

TABLE OF CONTENTS

Introduction...I

CHAPTER TWO: Snacks...1
   Avocado Roll-Ups..2
   Cucumber Bites..3
   No-Bake Oatmeal Bars..4
   Fruit Salad Skewers..5
   Pumpkin Pecan Granola Bars..6
   Baked Zucchini Fries with Garlic Aioli...7
   Roasted Sweet Potato Wedges with Cinnamon Sugar................8
   Cucumber Mint Water..9
   Honeydew Melon with Prosciutto..10
   Veggie Coconut Wraps...11
   Vegan Cashew Queso with Broccoli..12
   Chocolate Covered Banana Bites...13
   Stuffed Dates with Almond Butter...14
   Fruit and Veggie Smoothie...15
   Vegan Energy Balls...16
   Homemade Fruit Leather...17
   Healthy Caramel Pear Dip..18
   Apple Donuts...19
   Parmesan Zucchini Chips...20
   Mushroom Crostini With Herbs And Garlic................................21
   Roasted Beet Hummus with Carrot Sticks.................................22
   Cucumber Avocado Sushi Rolls..23
   Oven Baked Cinnamon Apple Chips..24
   Greek Yogurt with Honey and Berries..25
   Chia Seed Pudding with Almond Milk and Fresh Fruit...............26

CHAPTER THREE: Breakfasts...27
   Smashed Chickpea Bruschetta...28
   Tofu Scramble..29
   Cinnamon and Banana Porridge..30
   Mediterranean Breakfast Burrata...31
   Vegan Breakfast Burrito...32
   Low-Sugar Cranberry Orange Scones...33
   Breakfast Salad with Eggs..34

TABLE OF CONTENTS

Avocado Toast with Egg.....................35
Spicy Waffled Cauliflower Hash Browns.....................36
Sweet Potato, Bean, and Kale Shakshuka.....................37
Vanilla and Cinnamon Breakfast Rice.....................38
Overnight Oats with Strawberry and Passionfruit.....................39
Quinoa Breakfast Bowl with Peanut Butter and Banana.....................40
Chickpea Scramble with Tomato and Avocado.....................41
Sheet-Pan Vegan Sausage and Vegetables.....................42
Sweet Potato Banana Muffins.....................43
Butternut Squash Hash with Fried Eggs.....................45
Breakfast Loaded Sweet Potato.....................46
Watermelon and Berry Salad with Buckwheat.....................47
Whole Grain Pancakes With Cashew Butter.....................48
Fig, Nut, and Seed Bread with Ricotta and Fruit.....................49
Curried Chickpea Salad Wraps.....................51
Spicy Avocado Toasted Muffin with Shaved Ham and Spinach.....................52
Crunchy Oat Clusters with Peach and Yogurt.....................53
Quinoa Egg Muffins with Tomato, Basil and Mozzarella.....................54

CHAPTER FOUR: Lunches.....................55
Italian Panini with Provolone, Peppers, and Arugula.....................56
Curried Lentil Soup.....................57
Artichoke-Feta Quiche.....................58
Caprese Sandwich.....................60
Chicken Pot Stickers.....................61
Chopped Chicken and Broccoli Salad.....................62
Green Frittata.....................63
Mediterranean Chicken Wrap.....................64
Instant Pot Pakistani Chana Dal.....................65
Chicken Tortilla Soup.....................67
Chargrilled Lamb and Veggie Sandwich.....................68
Vegan Spinach and Sun-Dried Tomato Pasta.....................69
Asian Chicken Lettuce Wraps.....................70
Portobello Cheesesteak.....................71
Grilled Cheese and Tomato Soup.....................72
Pasta Salad with Lentils, Pesto, and Beans.....................73
Venezuelan Arepas with Black Beans.....................74

TABLE OF CONTENTS

Garlic Chili Chickpea Patties...75
Italian Tuna Melt..76
Gnocchi with Peas and Prosciutto...77
Minestrone with Pesto...78
Carne Asada Burritos..79
Chinese Garlic Tofu Stir Fry...80
Healthy Crab Cakes with Mango-Avocado Salsa..81
Dilled Salmon with Roasted Asparagus...83

CHAPTER FIVE: Dinners...84
Miso-Roasted Eggplant Steaks with Sweet Potatoes.....................................85
Chipotle Chicken Fajitas..86
Roasted Chicken and Potato With Kale Salad..88
Carrot Biryani..90
Curried Cod With Coconut Rice...91
Seared Tilapia With Spiralized Zucchini..92
Sheet-Pan Italian Pork Chops..93
Prawn, Fennel, and Asparagus Risotto..94
Chicken Teriyaki Bowls With Cauliflower Rice...95
Tempeh Lettuce Wraps...97
Creamy Chicken Quinoa Broccoli Casserole..98
Simple Sesame Chicken with Green Beans...100
Harissa and Citrus Baked Salmon...102
Vegan Chili..103
Rich Paprika Seafood Bowl..104
Avocado Soup..105
Summer Fish Stew..106
One Skillet Lemon Chicken and Bell Peppers and Spinach...........................107
Spiced Grilled Eggplant with Fresh Tomato Salad.......................................108
Moo Shu Mushroom Wraps...109
Chili-Stuffed Poblano Peppers..110
Sweet Potato & Bean Quesadillas...112
Roasted Cauliflower Tacos with Chipotle Cream...113
Broccoli Veggie Pasta Primavera...114
Seared Coconut Lime Chicken With Snap Pea Slaw.....................................115

TABLE OF CONTENTS

CHAPTER SIX: Desserts..116
Chocolate Chip Cookies..117
Lebanese Rice Pudding..118
New York Cheesecake..119
Blueberry Pie..120
Low-Fat Sugar-Free Key Lime Pie..121
Chocolate Pudding With Olive Oil and Sea Salt..122
Banana Bread..123
Tiramisu..124
Espresso Granita..125
Ricotta Cheesecake with Warm Blueberries..126
Brownie Cake Pops with Sprinkles..128
Chocolate-Dipped Fruit Pops..129
Frozen Yogurt Bark with Fruits and Nuts..130
Banana-Nutella Crepes..131
Savory and Sweet Olive Oil Ice Cream..132
Peach and Blueberry Greek Yogurt Cake..133
Fruit-Packed Mexican Paleta..134
Nectarine Blueberry Crisp..135
Grilled Pineapple with Vanilla Greek Yogurt..136
Roasted Strawberry Rhubarb Parfaits..137
Warm Banana Split in a Rum Sauce..138
Raspberry Coconut Oil Bites..139
Apple Nachos with Peanut Butter and Chocolate Sauce..140
Apple Turnovers..141
Peanut Butter & Chocolate Chickpea Blondies..142

TABLE OF CONTENTS

21-Day Meal Plan..143

Day 1:..144
Snack: Pumpkin Pecan Granola Bars..6
Breakfast: Cinnamon and Banana Porridge......................................30
Lunch: Venezuelan Arepas with Black Beans....................................74
Dinner: Vegan Chili..103
Dessert: Chocolate Chip Cookies...117

Day 2:..144
Snack: Veggie Coconut Wraps..11
Breakfast: Tofu Scramble...29
Lunch: Portobello Cheesesteak..71
Dinner: Chili-Stuffed Poblano Peppers...110
Dessert: Tiramisu...124

Day 3:..144
Snack: Baked Zucchini Fries with Garlic Aioli....................................7
Breakfast: Spicy Waffled Cauliflower Hash Browns..........................36
Lunch: Italian Tuna Melt...76
Dinner: Seared Coconut Lime Chicken With Snap Pea Slaw..........115
Dessert: Peach and Blueberry Greek Yogurt Cake...........................133

Day 4:..144
Snack: Fruit and Veggie Smoothie...15
Breakfast: Overnight Oats with Strawberry and Passionfruit.........39
Lunch: Minestrone with Pesto...78
Dinner: Sweet Potato & Bean Quesadillas...112
Dessert: Apple Nachos with Peanut Butter and Chocolate Sauce...140

Day 5:..145
Snack: Cucumber Avocado Sushi Rolls..24
Breakfast: Breakfast Loaded Sweet Potato.......................................46
Lunch: Gnocchi with Peas and Prosciutto..77
Dinner: Harissa and Citrus Baked Salmon...102
Dessert: Peanut Butter & Chocolate Chickpea Blondies..................142

TABLE OF CONTENTS

21-Day Meal Plan...143

Day 6:..145
Snack: Greek Yogurt with Honey and Berries.........................25
Breakfast: Fig, Nut, and Seed Bread with Ricotta and Fruit........49
Lunch: Grilled Cheese and Tomato Soup..............................72
Dinner: Chicken Teriyaki Bowls With Cauliflower Rice..............95
Dessert: Warm Banana Split in a Rum Sauce........................138

Day 7:..145
Snack: Oven Baked Cinnamon Apple Chips..........................24
Breakfast: Whole Grain Pancakes With Cashew Butter.............48
Lunch: Chicken Tortilla Soup...67
Dinner: Curried Cod With Coconut Rice...............................91
Dessert: Brownie Cake Pops with Sprinkles.........................128

Day 8:..145
Snack: Fruit Salad Skewers...5
Breakfast: Breakfast Salad with Eggs................................34
Lunch: Garlic Chili Chickpea Patties..................................75
Dinner: Sheet-Pan Italian Pork Chops................................93
Dessert: Espresso Granita..125

Day 9:..146
Snack: Avocado Roll-Ups..2
Breakfast: Butternut Squash Hash with Fried Eggs.................45
Lunch: Healthy Crab Cakes with Mango-Avocado Salsa...........81
Dinner: Chipotle Chicken Fajitas......................................86
Dessert: New York Cheesecake..119

Day 10:..146
Snack: Cucumber Bites..3
Breakfast: Quinoa Egg Muffins with Tomato, Basil and Mozzarella....54
Lunch: Dilled Salmon with Roasted Asparagus......................83
Dinner: Carrot Biryani..90
Dessert: Lebanese Rice Pudding.......................................118

TABLE OF CONTENTS

21-Day Meal Plan..143

Day 11:..146
Snack: Cucumber Mint Water...9
Breakfast: Smashed Chickpea Bruschetta...28
Lunch: Instant Pot Pakistani Chana Dal..65
Dinner: Prawn, Fennel, and Asparagus Risotto....................................94
Dessert: Fruit-Packed Mexican Paleta..134

Day 12:..146
Snack: Chocolate Covered Banana Bites...13
Breakfast: Mediterranean Breakfast Burrata..31
Lunch: Green Frittata..63
Dinner: Simple Sesame Chicken with Green Beans..............................100
Dessert: Grilled Pineapple with Vanilla Greek Yogurt..........................136

Day 13:..147
Snack: Healthy Caramel Pear Dip...18
Breakfast: Low-Sugar Cranberry Orange Scones...................................33
Lunch: Artichoke-Feta Quiche..58
Dinner: Rich Paprika Seafood Bowl..104
Dessert: Apple Turnovers..141

Day 14:..147
Snack: Vegan Energy Balls..16
Breakfast: Sweet Potato, Bean, and Kale Shakshuka............................37
Lunch: Italian Panini with Provolone, Peppers, and Arugula..................56
Dinner: Summer Fish Stew...106
Dessert: Raspberry Coconut Oil Bites..139

Day 15:..147
Snack: Apple Donuts...20
Breakfast: Sheet-Pan Vegan Sausage and Vegetables..........................42
Lunch: Caprese Sandwich..60
Dinner: Roasted Cauliflower Tacos with Chipotle Cream......................113
Dessert: Nectarine Blueberry Crisp..135

TABLE OF CONTENTS

21-Day Meal Plan..143

Day 16:..147
Snack: No-Bake Oatmeal Bars..4
Breakfast: Watermelon and Berry Salad with Buckwheat.................47
Lunch: Mediterranean Chicken Wrap...64
Dinner: Broccoli Veggie Pasta Primavera...................................114
Dessert: Frozen Yogurt Bark with Fruits and Nuts........................130

Day 17:..147
Snack: Roasted Sweet Potato Wedges with Cinnamon Sugar.............8
Breakfast: Crunchy Oat Clusters with Peach and Yogurt..................53
Lunch: Pasta Salad with Lentils, Pesto, and Beans........................73
Dinner: Spiced Grilled Eggplant with Fresh Tomato Salad...............108
Dessert: Chocolate Pudding With Olive Oil and Sea Salt..................122

Day 18:..148
Snack: Honeydew Melon with Prosciutto....................................10
Breakfast: Curried Chickpea Salad Wraps...................................51
Lunch: Carne Asada Burritos..79
Dinner: One Skillet Lemon Chicken and Bell Peppers and Spinach......107
Dessert: Low-Fat Sugar-Free Key Lime Pie..................................121

Day 19:..148
Snack: Vegan Cashew Queso with Broccoli..................................12
Breakfast: Sweet Potato Banana Muffins....................................43
Lunch: Chinese Garlic Tofu Stir Fry...80
Dinner: Creamy Chicken Quinoa Broccoli Casserole........................98
Dessert: Savory and Sweet Olive Oil Ice Cream............................132

Day 20:..148
Snack: Homemade Fruit Leather...17
Breakfast: Vegan Breakfast Burrito...32
Lunch: Chopped Chicken and Broccoli Salad.................................62
Dinner: Seared Tilapia With Spiralized Zucchini............................92
Dessert: Roasted Strawberry Rhubarb Parfaits.............................137

TABLE OF CONTENTS

21-Day Meal Plan..143

Day 21:...148
    Snack: Roasted Beet Hummus with Carrot Sticks..................................22
    Breakfast: Quinoa Breakfast Bowl with Peanut Butter and Banana............40
    Lunch: Curried Lentil Soup...57
    Dinner: Tempeh Lettuce Wraps...97
    Dessert: Banana-Nutella Crepes...131

About the Author..149
Index...151

CHAPTER ONE:

Introduction

INTRODUCTION

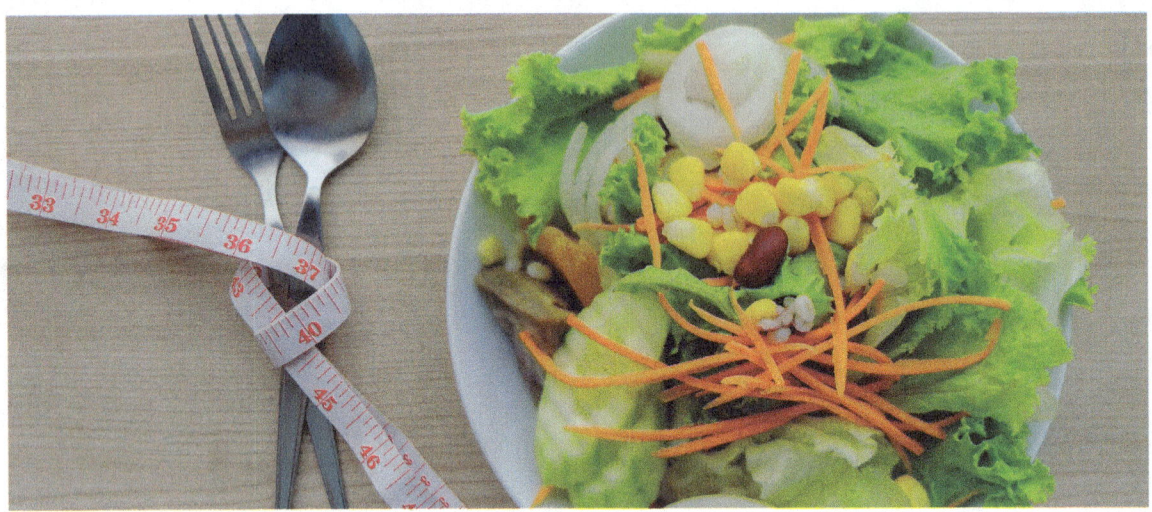

You've come to the right place. You're tired of picking up weight-loss cookbooks that make empty promises that don't work. Even worse are the ones that give you "guidance" that could actually be counterproductive to a healthy body and life. We understand completely, and that is why we made this book.

Healthy, natural weight loss isn't a fad. It's a goal toward leading a more comfortable, active, healthy life that makes you feel your happiest and most productive. Some people want to look better in a swimsuit, and others might want to lose weight for health reasons or to feel more at home in their own skin. For most of us, it's a combination of all valid and very personal reasons why we want to shed a few pounds and get back to doing the things we love to do, including eating the foods we love to eat.

This book is different. This book isn't going to try to kick the extra weight off with unnatural gimmicks or unhealthy suggestions. This cookbook you're holding in your hands is going to guide you toward a holistic, healthy lifestyle of eating well and feeling great while using foods' natural properties and your body's natural ability to burn calories to help you achieve your goals.

Over the past five years, obesity among adults has been estimated to have increased to nearly 33% of the population. That's a lot! It's no wonder that obesity-related health conditions are some of the leading causes of preventable death.

There are obviously a lot of reasons to want to maintain a healthy weight, and a lot of research to support why doing so is important. However, some ways of going about it are better than others. We're excited to show you that reaching and maintaining a healthy weight doesn't have to mean cutting calories.

You know that old saying, "Work smarter, not harder"? That's what we'd like to show you how to do for weight loss.

CALORIES CAN TAKE A BACKSEAT—FOOD IS THE REAL STAR OF THE SHOW

It's easy to fall back on the old-school idea that cutting calories is the best way to achieve weight loss. But in fact, research shows that the best way to achieve a healthy weight is to focus on feeding your body healthy foods and not counting calories.

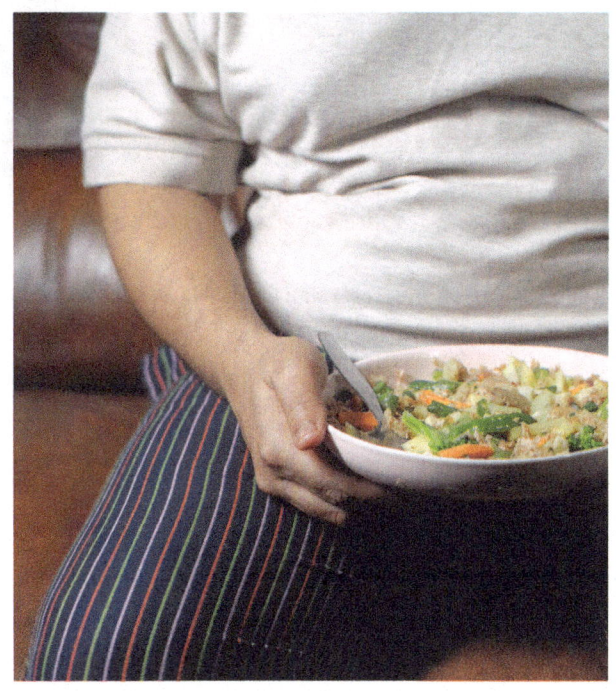

Becoming too obsessed with calorie counting can have a reverse effect on your health. Eating too little can put your health at risk by failing to provide the nutrients your body needs to function properly.

It can also lead to vitamin and mineral deficiencies that can cause a whole host of other health issues, some of which can be quite serious. Eating too few calories can cause your body to break down its very own tissue and muscle, making weight loss even more difficult by slowing your metabolic rate.

So, if your goal is to lose weight for a healthier life, why would you want to risk damaging your health to lose weight fast through artificial diet plans? Trust us, that's not the way to go. Instead, let's work toward a more effective and sustainable weight-loss plan, one that gives your body all the nutrients it needs while including food components that can naturally aid in weight loss. Eating whole, unprocessed, and high-quality foods can control your hunger and promote fat burning by increasing your metabolism. Doesn't that sound like a better idea already?

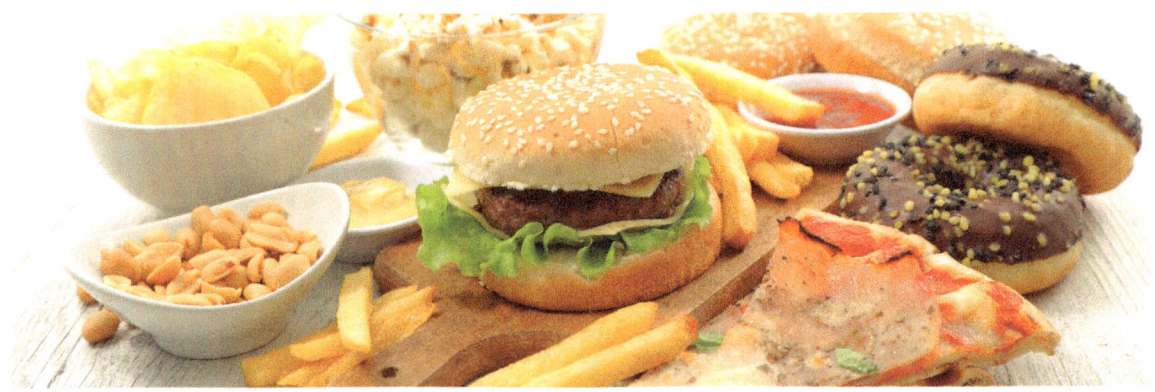

Sure, we all like to indulge from time to time on things like fried foods and refined sugars. But eating too many processed foods is a sure way to sabotage both your health and your weight. Overly processed foods are filled with ingredients that can sabotage your health, and they are also bad for your gut health. Good gut health can help decrease fat stored around your midsection and also decrease inflammation. It's also a lot easier to achieve your weight-loss goals when your gut is in tip-top shape.

You might be asking yourself, "If I don't start with calories, then where the heck do I start?" Good question, and we've got answers!

PLATE UP THE PROTEIN

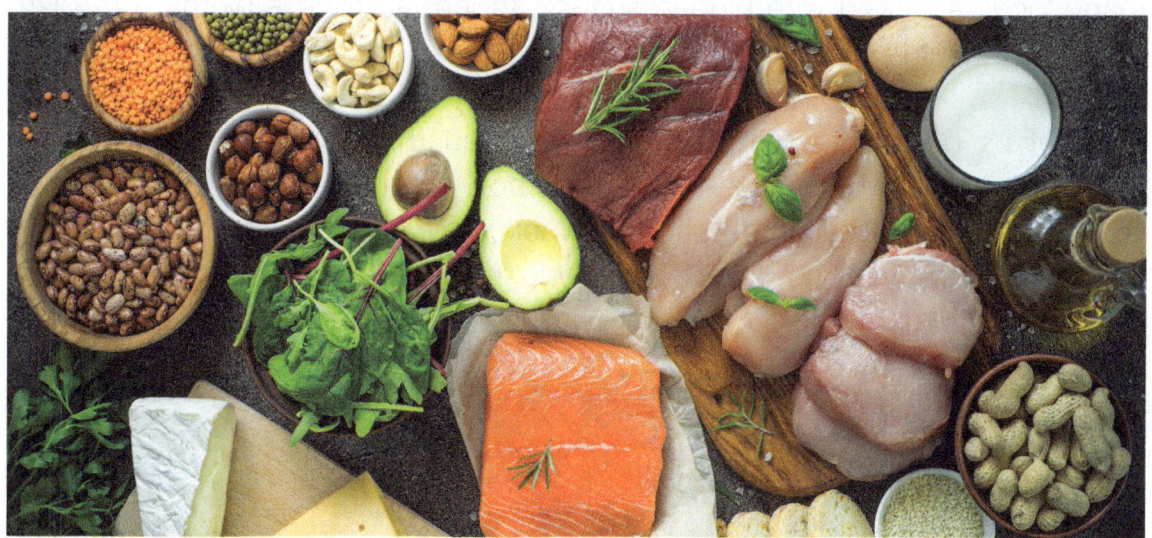

Protein tops the chart as far as nutrients go, especially when it comes to weight loss. Your body burns calories while it digests and metabolizes protein. So, it would make sense that a high-protein diet can boost your metabolism and increase fat-burning. It can also make you feel fuller and reduce your appetite when your diet is packed with protein.

One of nature's best-kept secrets is the egg—a simple, protein powerhouse that is low in calories, loaded with nutrients, and both easy and inexpensive to eat. Eating an egg for breakfast is a great start toward setting up your day for weight-loss success. It fills you up quickly and leaves you full for a while. Many meats contain protein like chicken, beef, and turkey, to name a few.

Just remember to try to keep your protein choices to lean proteins instead of fatty proteins. Salmon is not only high in protein but also in omega-3 fatty acids, which can keep you feeling fuller longer than other proteins. But for those vegans out there, no need to panic! Legumes, beans, and lentils are all rich in protein and contain the same healthy, calorie-burning benefits as their animal counterparts.

Another excellent thing you can do for both a healthy diet and natural weight loss is to build your diet on a foundation of whole, single-ingredient foods. So many foods are filled with hidden sugars, added fats, and a plethora of high-calorie ingredients in processed foods.

Most of us don't take the time to really read through every word on the ingredient labels, which makes it hard to know exactly what we're putting into our bodies. But when you choose whole, raw, unprocessed, and single-ingredient foods, you know exactly what you're eating, and you're skipping all the unnecessary junk.

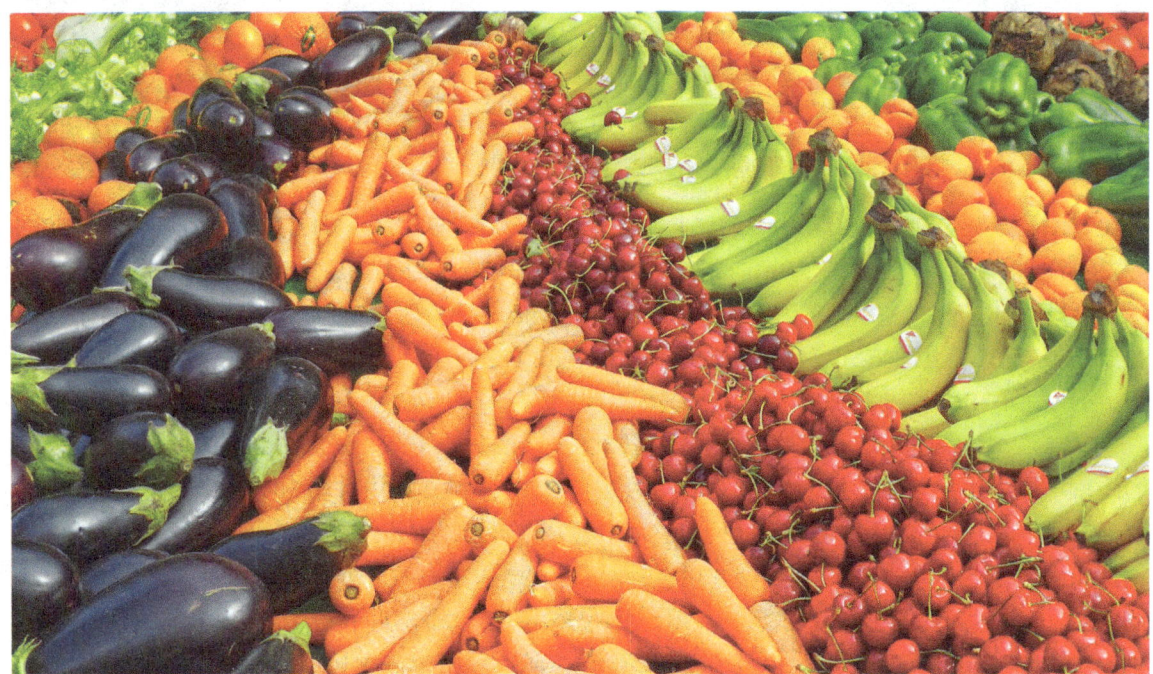

Many whole foods are naturally filling, providing your body with the essential nutrients it needs to work its best. Things like fruits and vegetables are very weight-loss-friendly, as natural foods are usually dense in water, nutrients, and fiber. Weight loss can be a natural side effect of eating whole foods and omitting processed ones without needing to count calories or spend hours reading through packaging labels.

Foods that are overly processed are low in nutrients and fiber and they're easy to digest, which means a spike in blood glucose levels and calories that settle into your fat cells quickly. When you eat a lot of them, the calories stored up in your fat cells continue to grow at a rate that is faster than what your body needs to pull energy from. Fortunately, there are no shortage of good alternatives out there to a bag of chips.

Nuts are great sources of fiber, protein, and healthy fats. They are also natural hunger suppressants. Avocados can also naturally decrease hunger as they are high in fiber. Most vegetables can assist natural weight loss as they are high in fiber and vitamins. Some, like dark leafy greens, are also good sources of protein. And that satisfying crunch from some vegetables can provide a satiating snack experience.

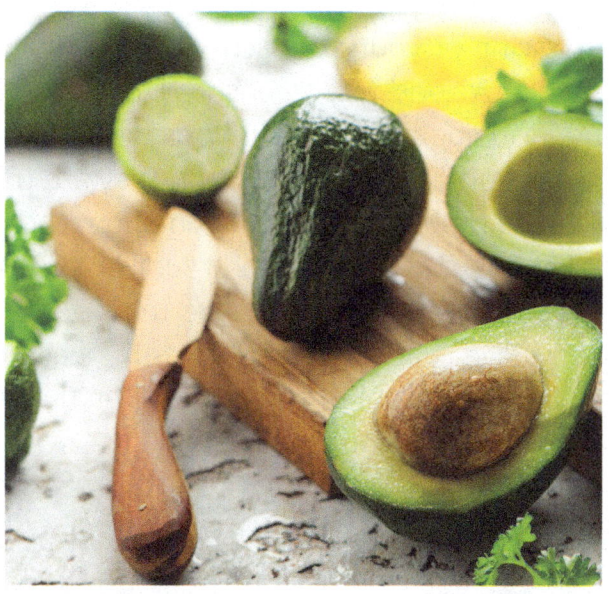

But there are also a few foods you might not have even thought about, like unripe bananas, which have one of the world's highest sources of prebiotic-resistant starch. This fiber-high substance can help prevent fat storage around your waistline.

Fiber-rich foods are helpful because they can keep you feeling fuller for longer. They naturally prompt you to eat less without you having to give it any thought or feel as if you are depriving yourself. Fiber is also good for your gut health, which, in turn, can reduce the risk of obesity. Dietary fiber slows digestion and helps regulate blood glucose levels, which then helps regulate insulin, a fat-storage hormone. Insulin can prevent you from overeating while also regulating and balancing your gut health and hormones.

Let's not forget about adding a little flavor and spice, which can also aid in weight loss. Chili peppers and jalapenos contain capsaicin, which can naturally reduce your appetite and boost metabolism. Also, chia seeds are a dual-purpose weight-loss warrior. They are packed with fiber to help you feel full and are also a natural appetite suppressant thanks to their nifty little trick of actually expanding in your stomach to take up more space after you eat them.

Speaking of your stomach, evidence suggests that gut bacteria may influence weight. A good way to ensure that your gut bacteria is balanced and healthy is by including probiotics in your diet. Probiotics are live bacteria found in foods like yogurt and kombucha, and they are useful in regulating healthy gut bacteria. They can also reduce inflammation and appetite. Although probiotics can be taken as a supplement, it's always best to get your nutrients from food whenever possible. In today's markets, there is a wide variety of products with active live cultures of probiotics in nearly every flavor of the rainbow. If you are lactose-intolerant or on a vegan diet, there are alternatives to meet your needs.

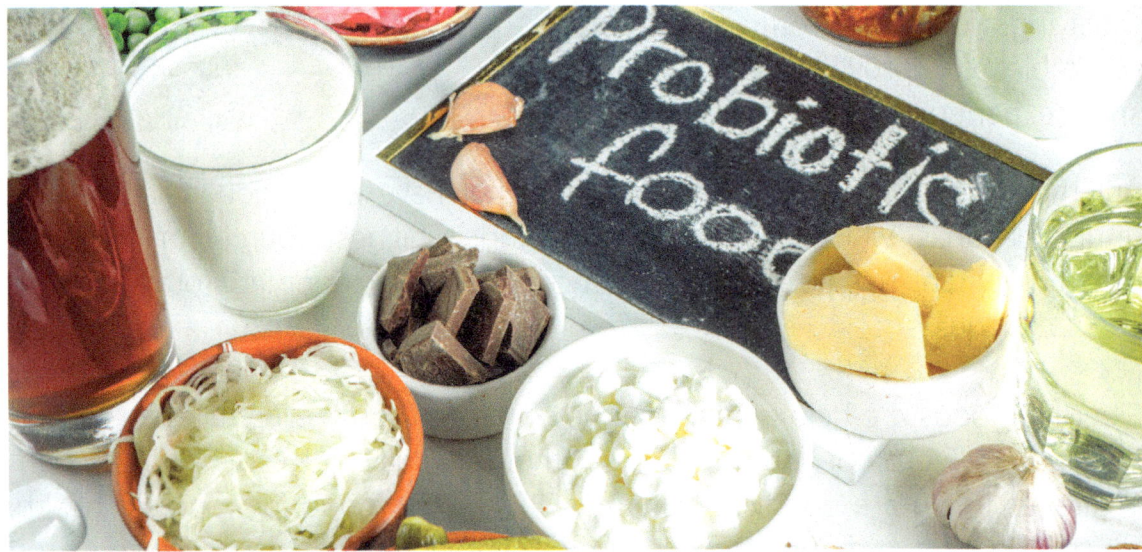

Now that we've spent some time talking about foods that can promote and help natural weight loss, let's change things up a bit and talk about something else you ingest every day—drinks.

TOP ME OFF PLEASE!

There are some beverages you probably don't want topped off if you are trying to reach and maintain a healthy weight, like alcohol or those sugar-loaded fancy lattes at the coffee shop. However, here are a couple of drinks that can help you take the weight off.

You don't have to order the tallest mocha frappe at the coffee shop; you can opt for something a bit simpler and a lot healthier. Black coffee actually has several important health benefits. It's loaded with antioxidants and can support weight loss by increasing energy levels. It can also boost your metabolism and make you feel full without ingesting hardly any calories at all.

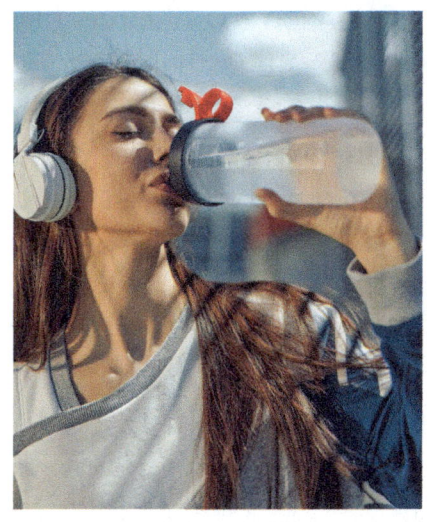

Yet, water is definitely top dog when it comes to aiding with weight loss above any other beverage you might consume. Drinking water can increase the calories you burn and can also lead to reduced calorie intake if you drink water before your meals. And when you replace other drinks high in calories or sugar with a glass of water, you are avoiding the empty calories you may have otherwise consumed. Your body needs water in order to function properly, and staying well-hydrated is critical for your metabolism.

If you're not a big fan of drinking plain water, you can infuse your water bottle with mint or cucumber. Doing so will add both taste and healthy properties that can benefit you in multiple ways at once.

With the right food and beverage choices, you're off to a great start for both weight loss and optimal health. Now, let's engage a few other components to a lifestyle that supports a healthy weight before we delve into the delicious dishes in this book!

MINDFUL MEALS

Sometimes, it's about how you think and feel that make the most difference. Your relationship with food is no different. If you feel like you are depriving yourself, your diet won't be sustainable. But if you feel like you can still enjoy your meals and have the things you want in moderation—and if you look at these healthy lifestyle changes as a path to a healthier, happier you—then you are more apt to embrace what you are doing. Sometimes, all we need is a little tip or trick to turn the tables and get our head fully on board.

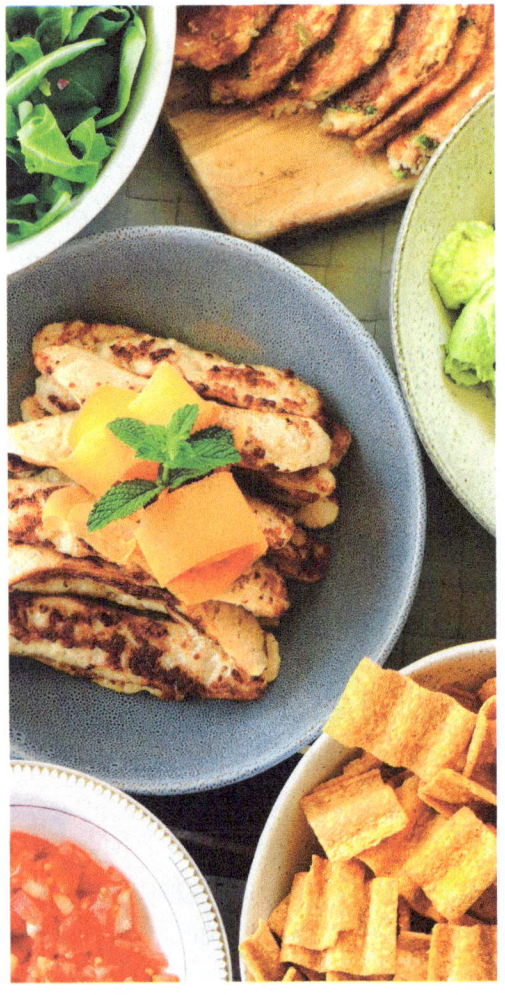

One major tip is to practice mindful eating. Mindful eating increases your awareness while you are enjoying your food. It involves paying attention to your body to recognize when you are actually hungry versus when you are just bored. Therefore, mindful eating can help you make good food choices while preventing stress and binge-eating.

Smaller plate sizes can also help. People can get into the habit of eating what is on their plate in front of them. They can also get into the habit of filling a plate regardless of its size. So, take a minute to choose the right size that truly matches your hunger. Then, while you're eating it, be mindful of the tastes, smells, and presentation of your food. Enjoy your meal instead of just piling on a forkful. Doing so will help you slow down and digest well, and really be able to tell when you feel full.

Along with mindful meals comes mindful physical activity. Exercise is a great component to a healthy lifestyle and an integral part to managing a healthy weight. There are endless options to the types of exercise you can do, ranging from low to high-impact, beginner to advanced levels, and indoor or outdoor activities. Just be sure you feed your body with good nutrition that balances your physical exertion. You can't pull from an empty tank.

If you want your body to perform at its best and work efficiently to shed excess weight, you must provide it with the proper nutrition to do so. Protect those muscles with lots of good proteins, hydrate well to offset loss of fluids with sweat, and find an exercise regimen you enjoy so that you are more likely to stick with it.

Exercise, like food, should be enjoyable. If you hate running, then don't run. If you are bored by sitting on a stationary bike, don't get on one. Try a barre class or an online ballet video or go for a walk through the city in the cool air. There is no one set exercise or diet that will be the perfect fit for everyone. You need to find and choose what is good for you—what makes you feel good physically and makes you happy.

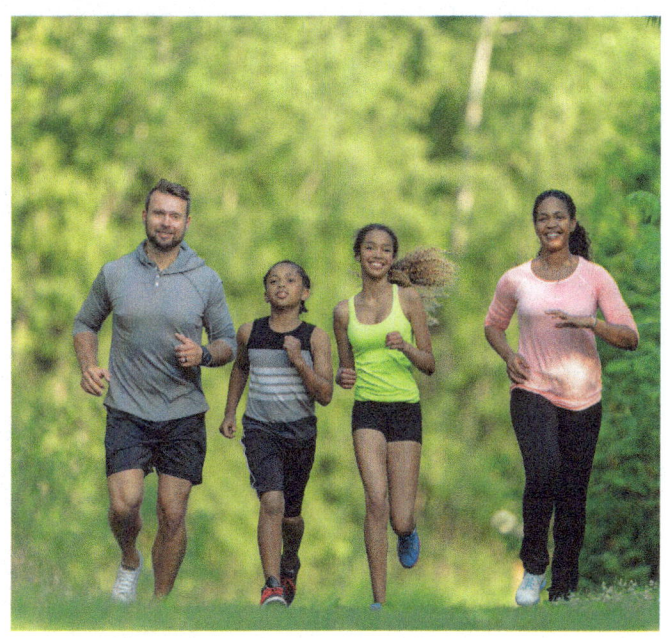

There's one thing we know will make you happy—the recipes in this book! We've compiled our expertise to collect a stunning array of recipes for you. After all, you're busy moving and shaking, getting ready to reach your lifestyle and weight loss goals. So, we thought we'd step in and take the guesswork out of meal prep so that you can get right on your way to healthy eating.

The recipes in this cookbook center on the principles of natural, holistic weight loss. It features foods that are already good for you while having the added benefit of naturally enhancing weight-loss properties. We've chosen all the best ingredients and made sure that they are things you won't have a hard time looking for in the store.

We've provided you with simple instructions that will make meal prep a breeze, leaving you more time to do all the things you love. And the best part of all is that each and every dish in this book is designed to be delicious!

Sure, we've made sure everything is conducive to achieving a healthy weight. But we've also made sure that your tastebuds won't suffer in the process! The dishes on the following pages are so tempting, you won't feel like you're missing out on anything at all! In fact, you might find yourself feeling like you've never eaten so well in your life!

And if there happens to be a recipe or ingredient that doesn't make you swoon with delight, we've also made sure to provide easy alternatives and make the dishes highly modifiable so that you can tweak them to your own tastes.

Part of losing weight the natural way and staying at a healthy weight healthy is ensuring that the lifestyle choices you make are sustainable for the long term. To that end, you need to have food that you want to eat and enjoy—and boy, do we have you covered for that!

All you need to do is choose a recipe that looks intriguing and appealing to you, then follow the simple directions that will walk you through creating a culinary masterpiece.

And when the dish is done, and you find yourself savoring a tasty new meal, take a mindful moment to think about all the ways these foods are helping your body to be in optimal shape so that it can support a long, happy, and healthy life.

Food is your friend, not your foe, and that is especially true for weight loss. So, say goodbye to all of those restricting diet fads or the notion that food is the culprit behind unhealthy weight gain—nothing could be farther from the truth.

Nourishing, healthy, and delicious foods are necessary for your beautiful body, and are also part of life's joys. Healthy weight management and responsible, natural weight loss are positive and enjoyable experiences you can now look at in a whole new light thanks to all that you have learned, and thanks to this book brimming with wonderful new meal creations.

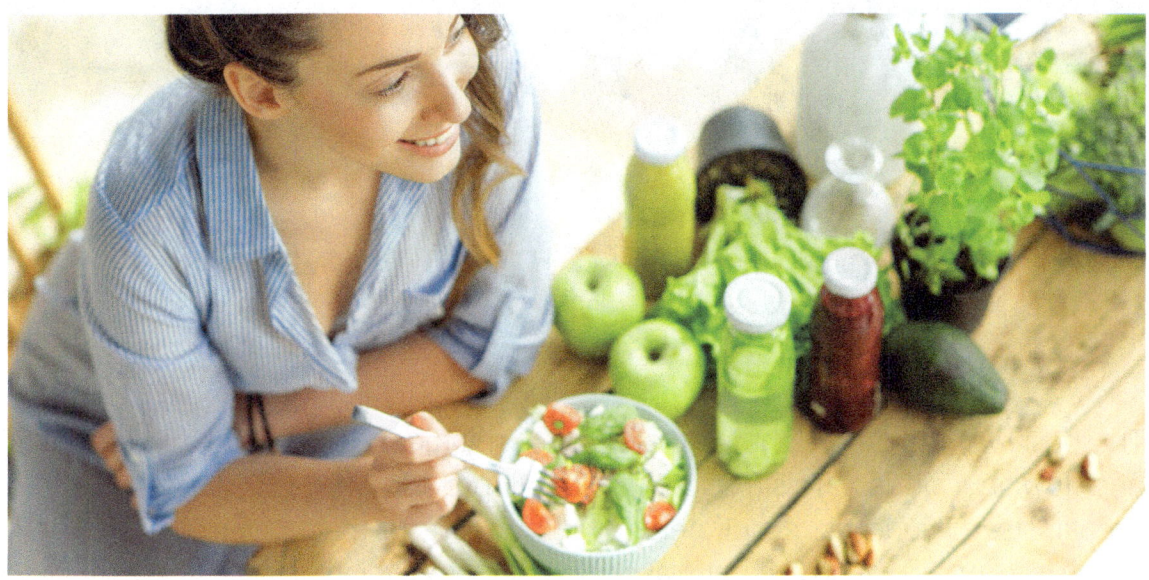

Go ahead and indulge in everything this cookbook has to offer because while you're at it, your body will be hard at work shedding weight the way it was designed to do.

HEALTHY RECIPES FOR WEIGHT LOSS

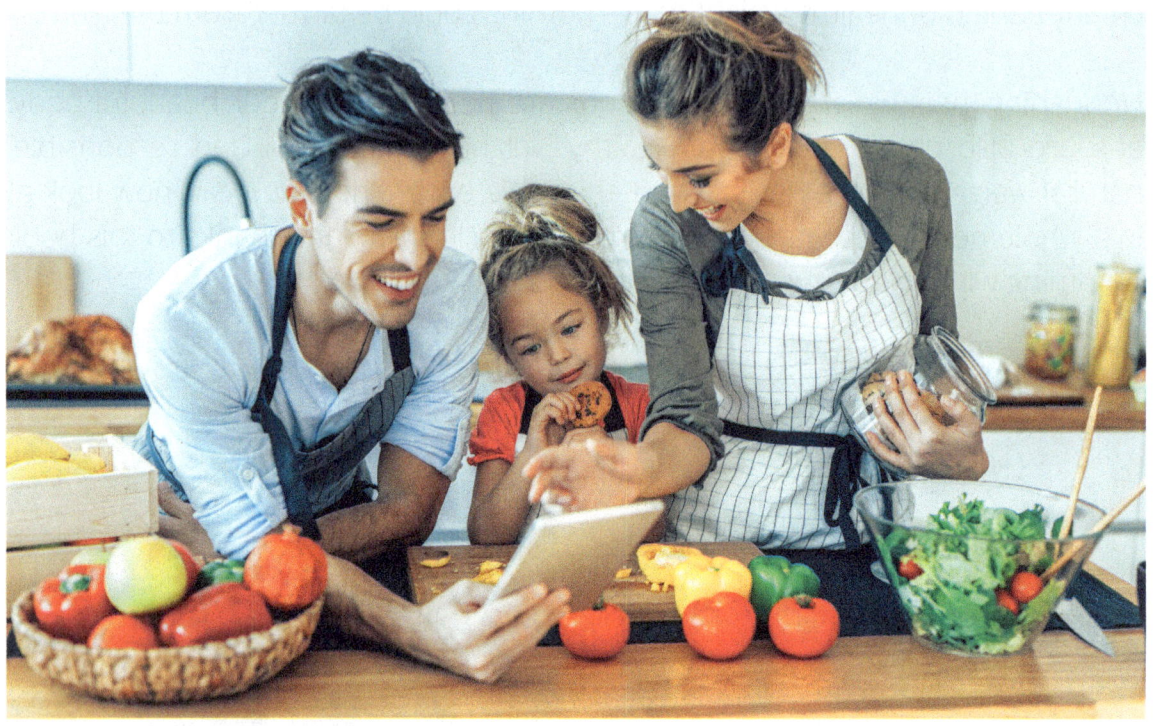

The best way to lose weight is by eating healthy meals that are rich in nutrients and low in calories. This recipe book will provide you with 25 snacks, 25 breakfasts, 25 lunches, 25 dinners, and 25 desserts that are healthy, natural, sugar-free, organic, and are neutral or beneficial for weight loss.

Each recipe includes:
- Ingredients
- Instructions
- Serving size
- Calories

So what are you waiting for? Start cooking up these delicious and nutritious meals today!

CHAPTER TWO:

Snacks

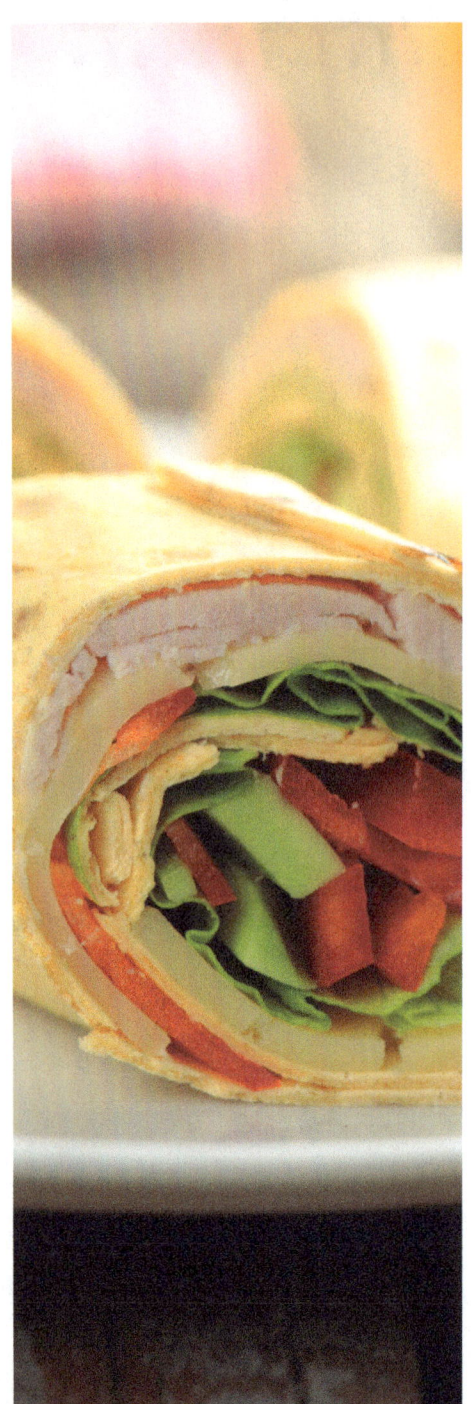

AVOCADO ROLL-UPS

Ingredients:

- 4 small whole wheat tortillas
- 1 ripe avocado, diced
- 1/4 cup finely diced red onion
- 1/4 cup finely diced red bell pepper
- 1/4 cup finely diced yellow bell pepper
- 1/4 cup finely diced green bell pepper
- Salt (optional) and black pepper (optional) to taste

Instructions:

1. Preheat oven to 350 degrees F.
2. In a medium bowl, mix together all of the ingredients for the filling.
3. Lay out each tortilla on a flat surface. Spread 1/2 of the filling evenly over each tortilla, leaving a 1-inch border around the edges. Roll up each tortilla tightly, burrito-style.
4. Place on a greased baking sheet and bake for 15-20 minutes, or until tortillas are crispy. Serve immediately!

Serving Size: 1 roll-up
Calories: 150

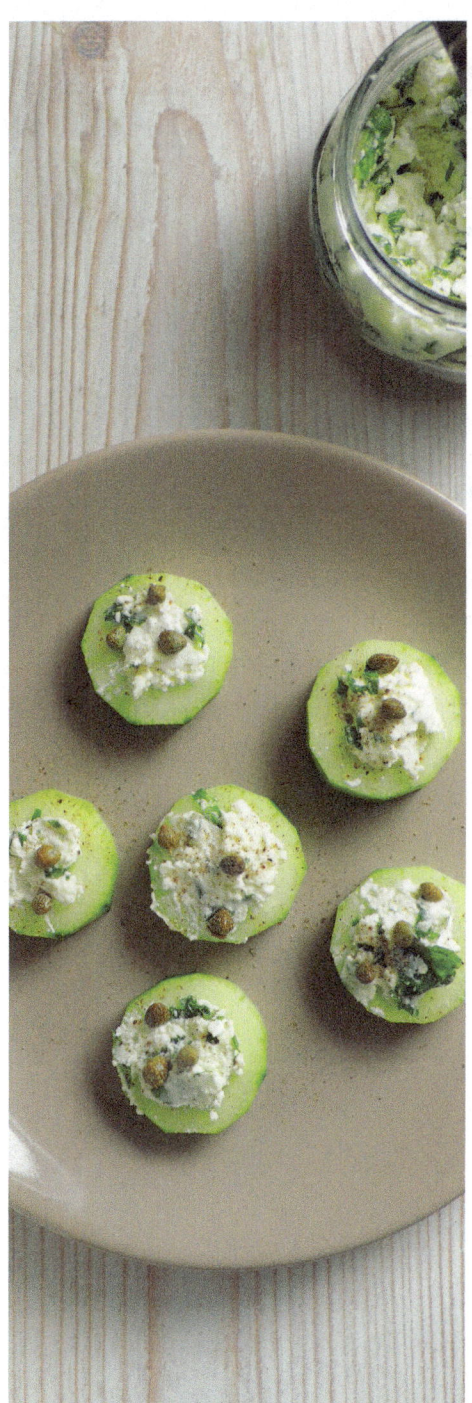

CUCUMBER BITES

Ingredients:
- 1 large cucumber, sliced into rounds
- 1/4 cup vegan cream cheese
- 1/4 cup shredded dairy-free cheese
- Salt (optional) and black pepper (optional) to taste

Instructions:
1. Preheat oven to 375 degrees F.
2. In a small bowl, mix together vegan cream cheese, shredded cheese, salt, and black pepper (optional).
3. Spread 1 teaspoon of the mixture onto each cucumber round.
4. Place on a greased baking sheet and bake for 10-15 minutes, or until cheese is melted and bubbly. Serve immediately!

Serving Size: 1 bite
Calories: 25

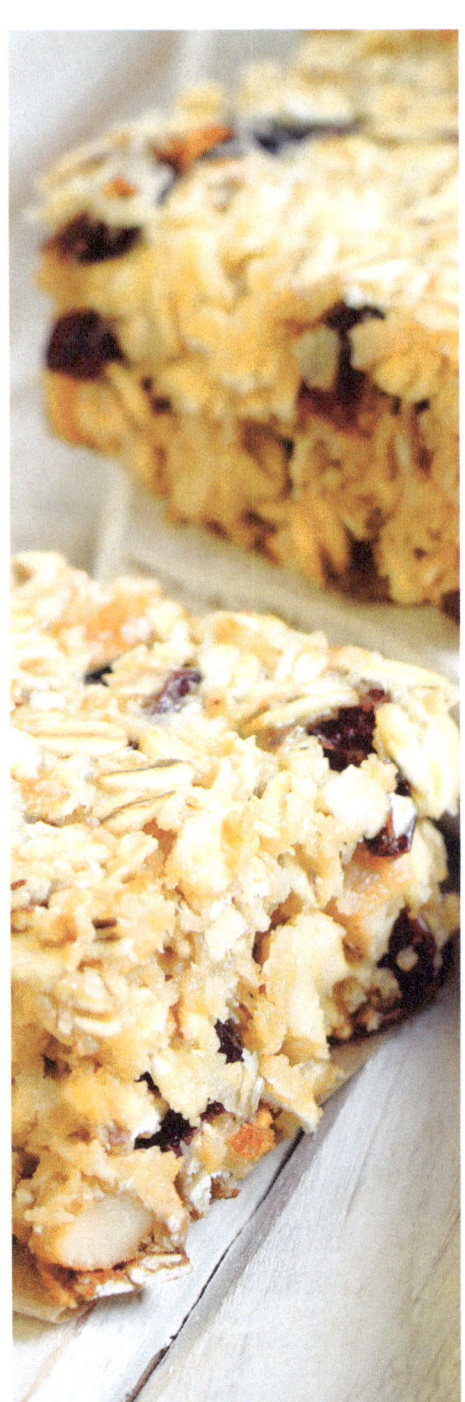

NO-BAKE OATMEAL BARS

Ingredients:
- 1 cup quick-cooking oats
- 1/2 cup finely diced dried fruit
- 1/4 cup finely chopped nuts
- 1/4 cup natural peanut butter

Instructions:
1. In a medium bowl, mix together all of the ingredients for the filling.
2. Grease an 8x8 inch baking dish and spread mixture evenly into the dish. Cover with plastic wrap and refrigerate for 30 minutes, or until firm. Cut into bars and serve immediately!

Serving Size: 1 bar
Calories: 210

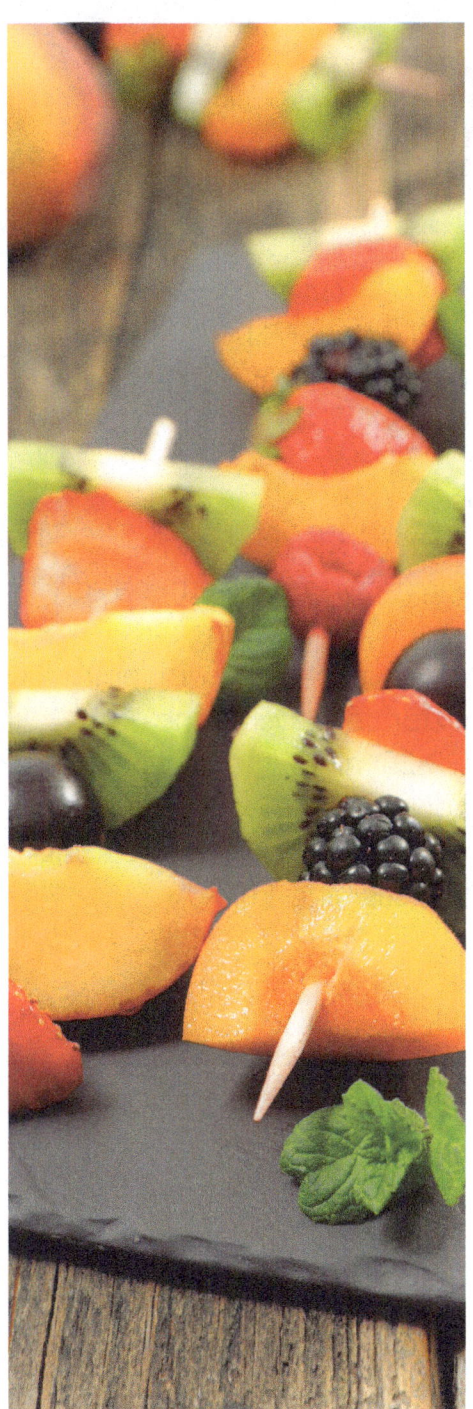

FRUIT SALAD SKEWERS

Ingredients:
- 1 large cantaloupe, cut into bite-sized chunks
- 1 large honeydew melon, cut into bite-sized chunks
- 1 large watermelon, cut into bite-sized chunks
- 1 pint fresh strawberries, hulled and halved

Instructions:
1. If using wooden skewers, soak in water for 30 minutes before assembly.
2. Alternate cantaloupe, honeydew, watermelon, and strawberries on each skewer. Serve immediately!

Serving Size: 1 skewer
Calories: 25

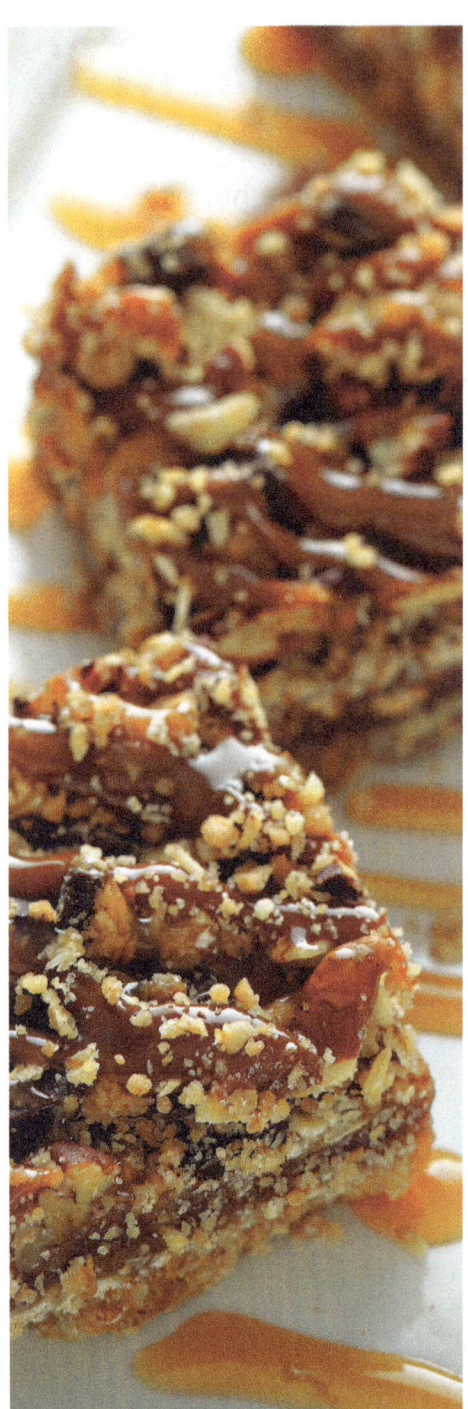

PUMPKIN PECAN GRANOLA BARS

Ingredients:
- 1 1/2 cups quick-cooking oats
- 1/2 cup finely chopped pecans
- 1/4 cup pumpkin puree
- 1/4 cup honey

Instructions:
1. Preheat oven to 375 degrees F.
2. In a medium bowl, mix together all of the ingredients for the filling.
3. Grease an 8x8 inch baking dish and spread mixture evenly into the dish. Bake for 20-25 minutes, or until bars are golden brown and firm to the touch. Allow to cool completely before cutting into bars and serving. Enjoy!

Serving Size: 1 bar
Calories: 210

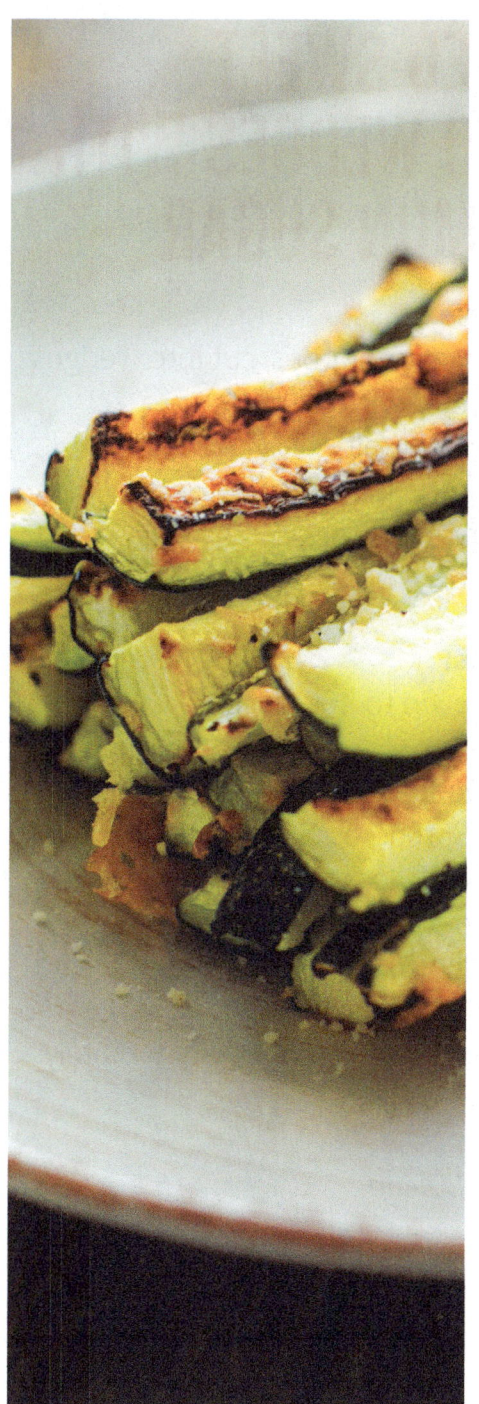

BAKED ZUCCHINI FRIES WITH GARLIC AIOLI

Ingredients:
- 1 large zucchini, cut into fry-sized sticks
- 1/2 cup whole wheat flour
- 1/4 teaspoon salt
- 1/4 teaspoon black pepper
- 1/2 cup non-dairy milk

For the garlic aioli:
- 1/4 cup vegan mayonnaise
- 2 cloves garlic, minced

Instructions:
1. Preheat oven to 400 degrees F.
2. In a large bowl, mix together flour, salt, and pepper.
3. Dip zucchini sticks into the milk mixture, then coat with the flour mixture. Place on a greased baking sheet.
4. Bake for 20-25 minutes, or until golden brown and crispy.
5. While zucchini fries are baking, prepare the garlic aioli by mixing together vegan mayonnaise and minced garlic in a small bowl. Serve immediately with zucchini fries!

Serving Size: 1/2 cup
Calories: 190

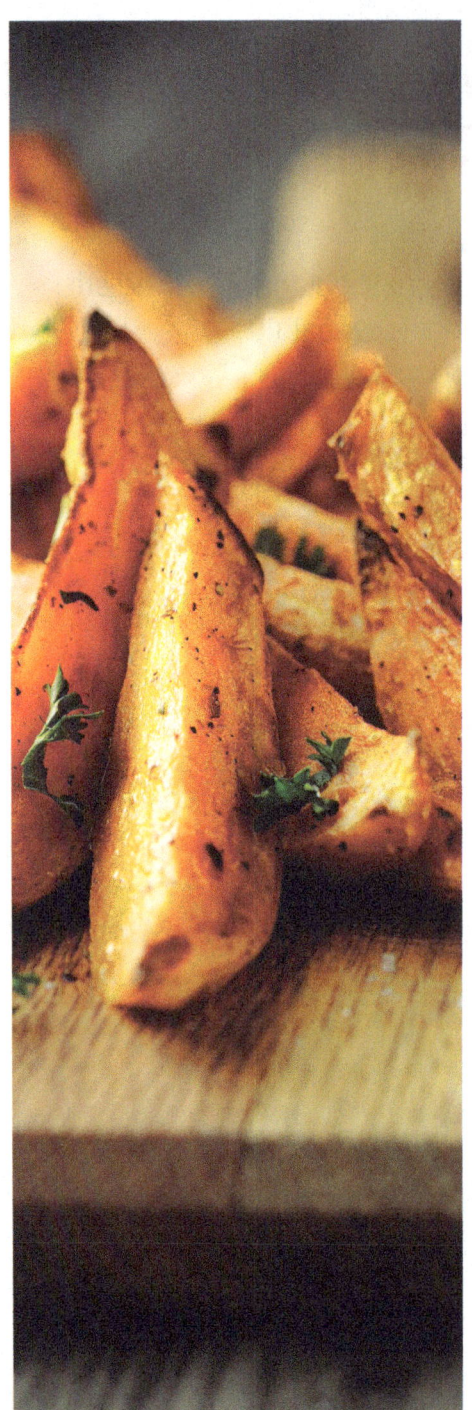

ROASTED SWEET POTATO WEDGES WITH CINNAMON SUGAR

Ingredients:
- 2 large sweet potatoes, cut into wedges
- 1 tablespoon olive oil
- 1/4 teaspoon salt
- 1/4 teaspoon black pepper
- 1 tablespoon sugar
- 1 teaspoon ground cinnamon

Instructions:
1. Preheat oven to 400 degrees F.
2. In a large bowl, toss together sweet potato wedges, olive oil, salt, and black pepper. Spread on a greased baking sheet and bake for 20-25 minutes, or until tender.
3. In a small bowl, mix together sugar and ground cinnamon. Sprinkle over roasted sweet potatoes and serve immediately!

Serving Size: 1/2 cup
Calories: 120

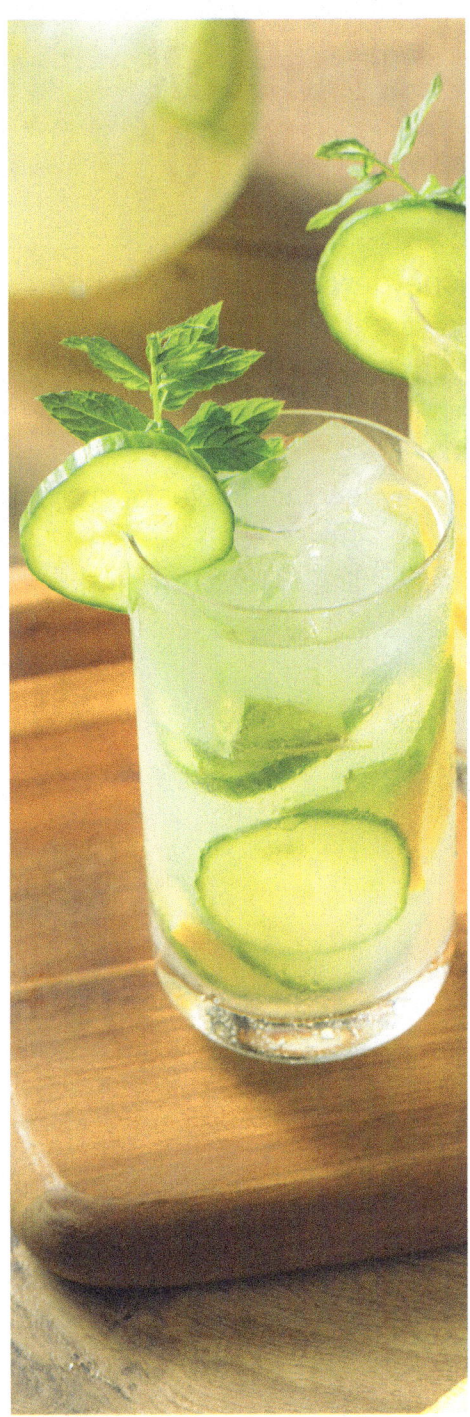

CUCUMBER MINT WATER

Ingredients:
- 1 large cucumber, thinly sliced
- 1/2 bunch fresh mint leaves
- 1/2 lemon, thinly sliced
- 1 gallon filtered water

Instructions:
1. Combine all ingredients in a large pitcher or container. Allow to steep overnight in the refrigerator.
2. Serve over ice and enjoy!

Serving Size: 1 cup
Calories: 0

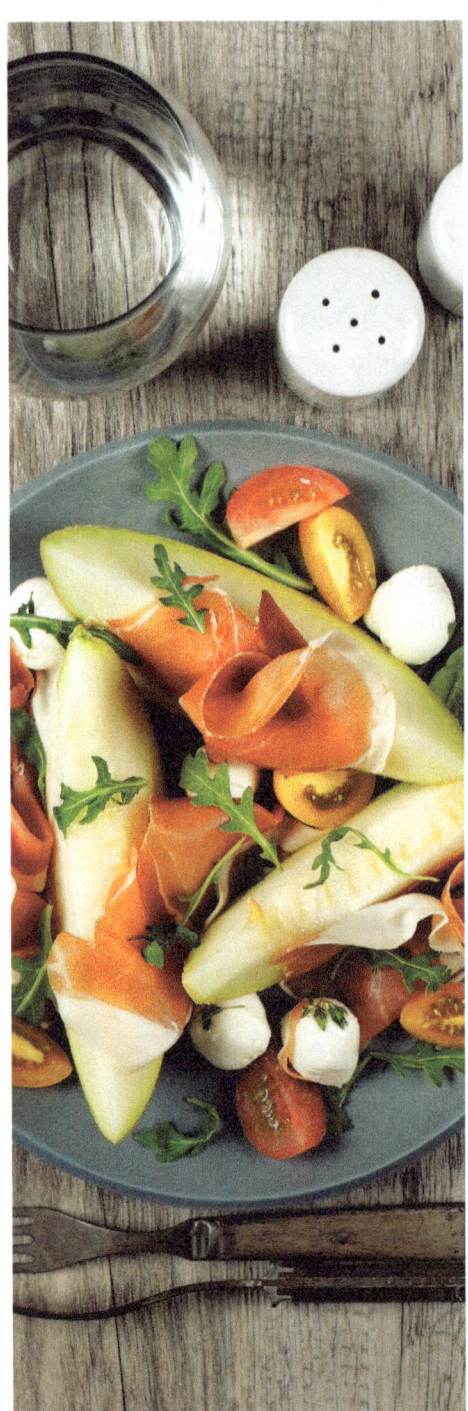

HONEYDEW MELON WITH PROSCIUTTO

Ingredients:

- 1 small honeydew melon, cut into bite-sized pieces
- 4 ounces thinly sliced prosciutto

Instructions:

1. Arrange honeydew melon pieces on a plate.
2. Top with thinly sliced prosciutto and serve immediately!

Serving Size: 1/2 cup
Calories: 120

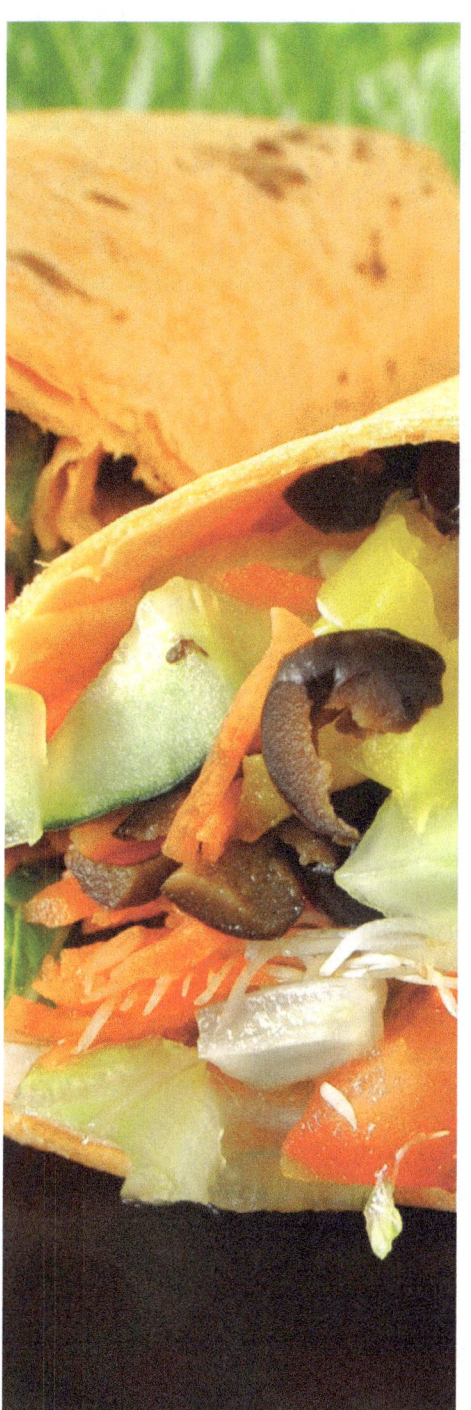

VEGGIE COCONUT WRAPS

Ingredients:
- 4 large lettuce leaves
- 1/2 cup shredded carrots
- 1/2 cup diced cucumber
- 1/4 cup chopped fresh cilantro
- 1/4 cup diced avocado

For the sauce:
- 1/4 cup diced mango
- 1 tablespoon lime juice
- 1 tablespoon finely chopped fresh ginger

Instructions:
1. In a small bowl, mix together all of the ingredients for the sauce. Set aside.
2. Place lettuce leaves on a plate and top with shredded carrots, diced cucumber, cilantro, and avocado. Drizzle with sauce and enjoy!

Serving Size: 1 wrap
Calories: 210

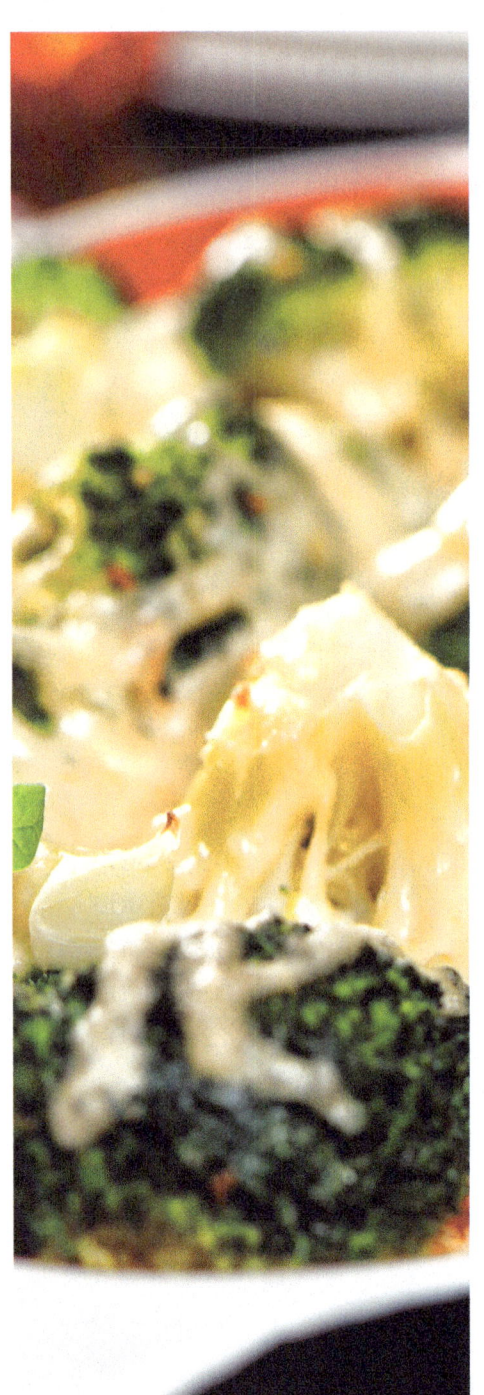

VEGAN CASHEW QUESO WITH BROCCOLI

Ingredients:
- 1 cup raw cashews, soaked for at least 2 hours
- 1/4 cup nutritional yeast flakes
- 1/2 teaspoon garlic powder
- 1/2 teaspoon onion powder
- 1/4 teaspoon chili powder
- 1 cup broccoli florets

Instructions:
1. Preheat oven to 350 degrees F.
2. In a food processor, combine all of the ingredients for the queso and blend until smooth and creamy.
3. Spread queso on a greased baking dish and top with broccoli florets. Bake for 10-15 minutes, or until broccoli is tender and queso is hot and bubbly. Serve immediately!

Serving Size: 1/4 cup
Calories: 120

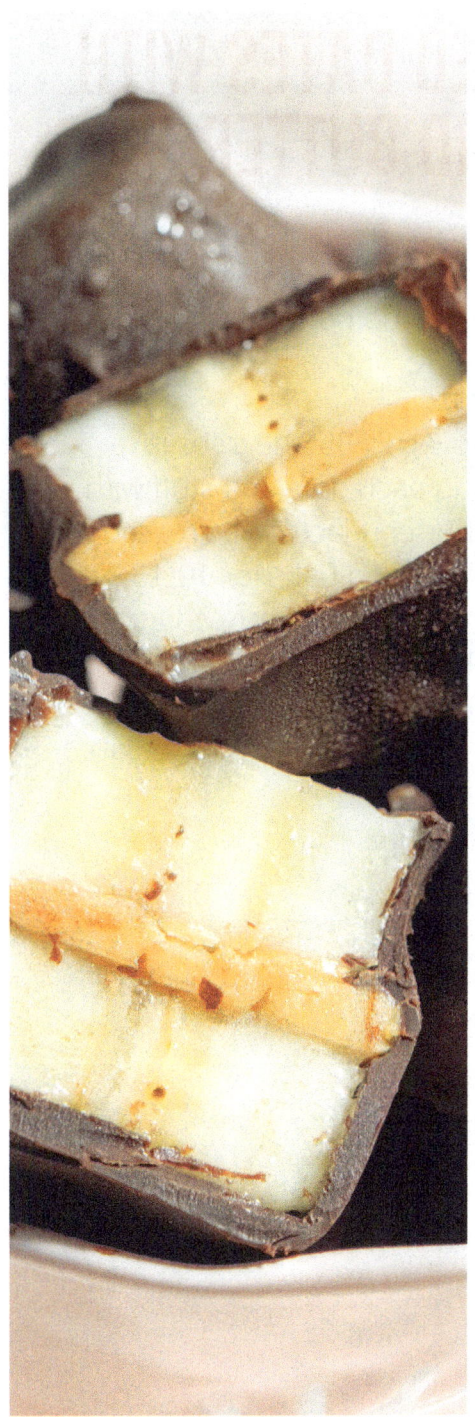

CHOCOLATE COVERED BANANA BITES

Ingredients:
- 1 large banana, cut into bite-sized pieces
- 1/4 cup vegan chocolate chips

Instructions:
1. Place banana bites on a plate or in a bowl.
2. Melt vegan chocolate chips in a double boiler or in the microwave. Drizzle over banana bites and enjoy!

Serving Size: 1/4 cup
Calories: 120

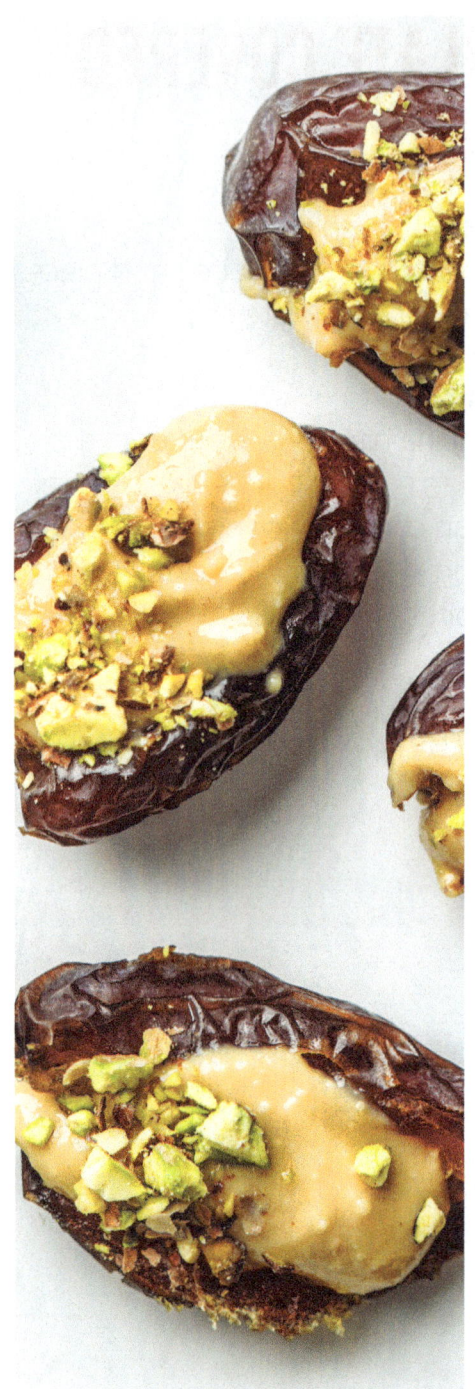

STUFFED DATES WITH ALMOND BUTTER

Ingredients:
- 12 large dates, pitted
- 1/4 cup almond butter

Instructions:
1. Preheat oven to 350 degrees F.
2. Cut a slit in each date and stuff with almond butter. Place on a greased baking sheet and bake for 10-15 minutes, or until dates are soft and almond butter is melted. Serve immediately!

Serving Size: 1 date
1. Calories: 100

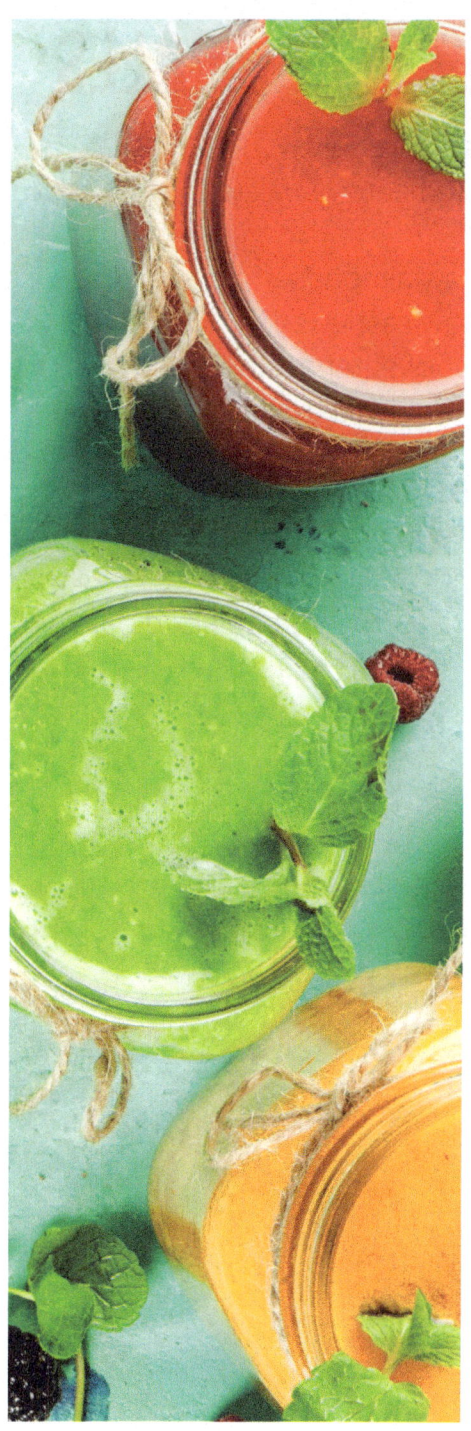

FRUIT AND VEGGIE SMOOTHIE

Ingredients:
- 1 cup frozen mixed berries
- 1/2 ripe banana
- 1/2 cup chopped kale or spinach
- 1/2 cup unsweetened almond milk

Instructions:
1. Place all ingredients in a blender and blend until smooth and creamy. Enjoy immediately!

Serving Size: 1 cup
Calories: 160

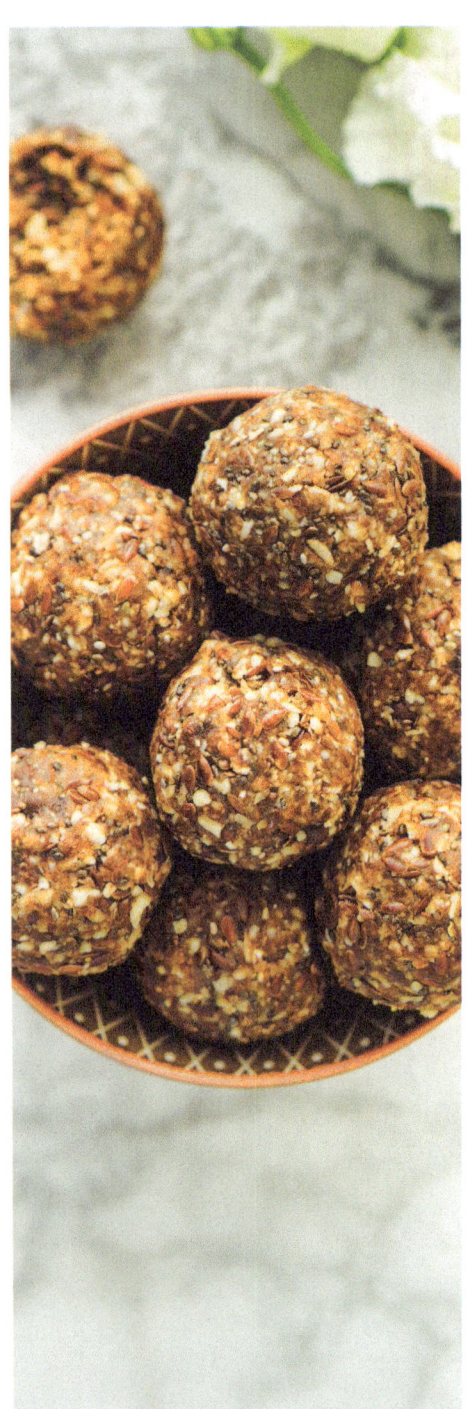

VEGAN ENERGY BALLS

Ingredients:
- 1 cup pitted dates, soaked for at least 2 hours
- 1/4 cup raw almonds
- 1/4 cup raw cashews
- 1/4 cup unsweetened shredded coconut
- 1 teaspoon vanilla extract

Instructions:
1. In a food processor, combine all of the ingredients and blend until well combined. Form into bite-sized balls and enjoy!

Serving Size: 1 ball
Calories: 100

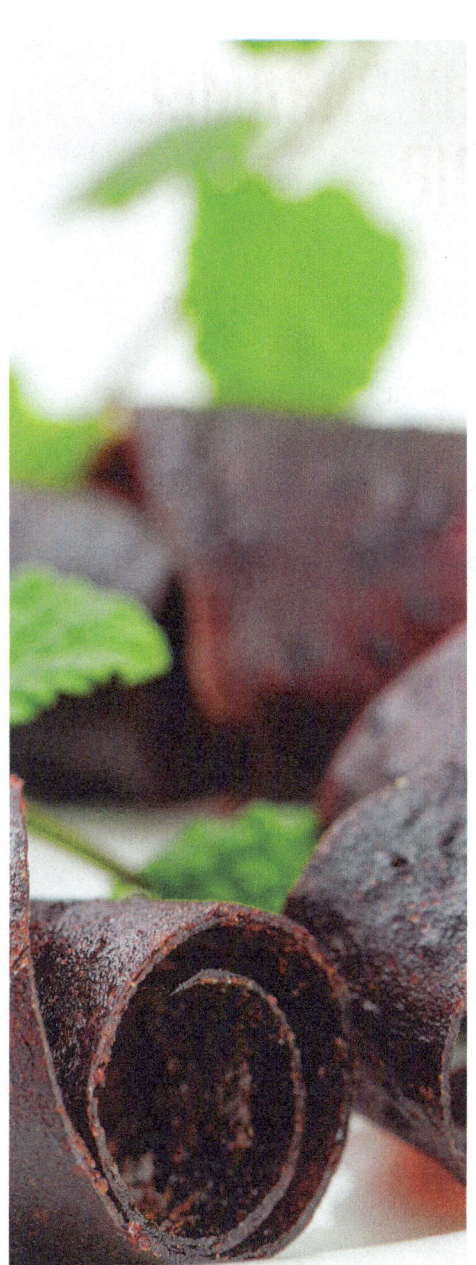

HOMEMADE FRUIT LEATHER

Ingredients:
- 1 cup pureed fruit (strawberries, raspberries, or applesauce)

Instructions:
1. Preheat oven to 200 degrees F.
2. Line a baking sheet with parchment paper and spread fruit puree evenly over the surface. Bake for 6-8 hours, or until leather is dry and slightly sticky to the touch. Allow to cool completely before cutting into strips. Enjoy!

Serving Size: 1 strip
Calories: 60

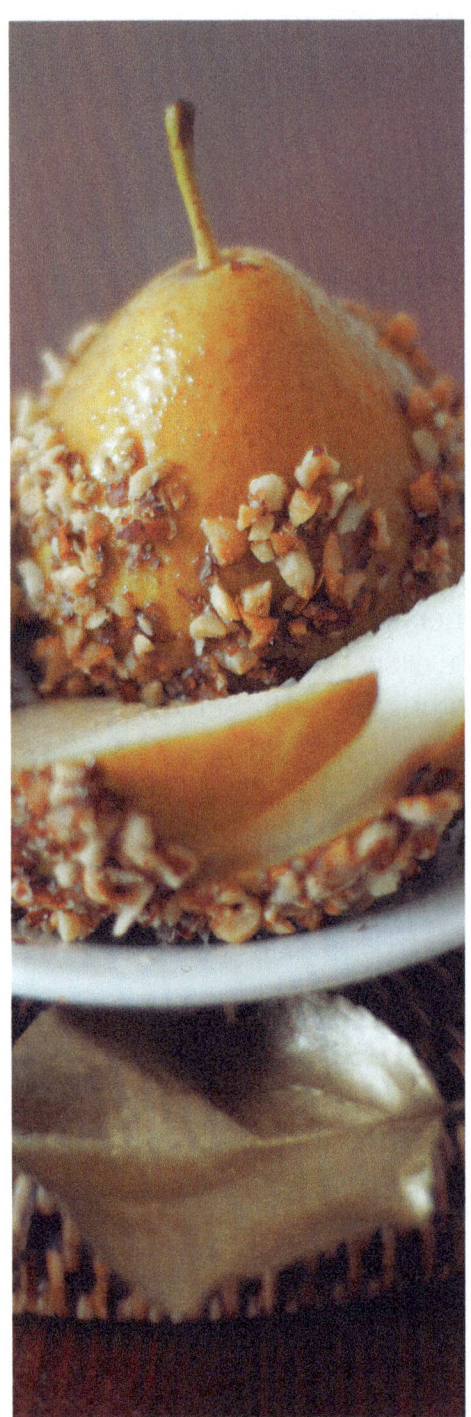

HEALTHY CARAMEL PEAR DIP

Ingredients:
- 1 large pear, peeled and diced

For the caramel dip:
- 1/4 cup almond butter
- 1 tablespoon maple syrup

Instructions:
1. In a small bowl, mix together all of the ingredients for the caramel dip. Set aside.
2. Place diced pear in a serving dish and top with caramel dip. Serve immediately!

Serving Size: 1/4 cup
Calories: 150

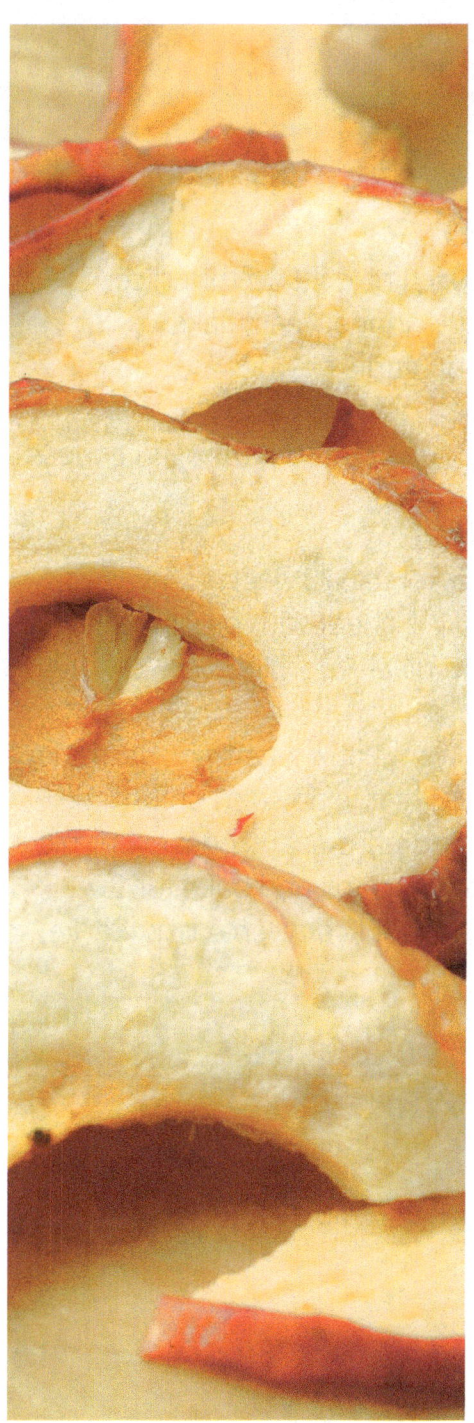

APPLE DONUTS

Ingredients:
- 1 large apple, cut into thin slices

For the topping:
- 1/4 cup vegan chocolate chips
- 1 tablespoon unsweetened shredded coconut

Instructions:
1. Preheat oven to 350 degrees F.
2. Line a baking sheet with parchment paper and place apple slices on the surface.
3. Melt vegan chocolate chips in a double boiler or in the microwave. Drizzle over apples and top with shredded coconut. Bake for 10-15 minutes, or until apples are soft and chocolate is melted. Serve immediately!

Serving Size: 1 donut
Calories: 100

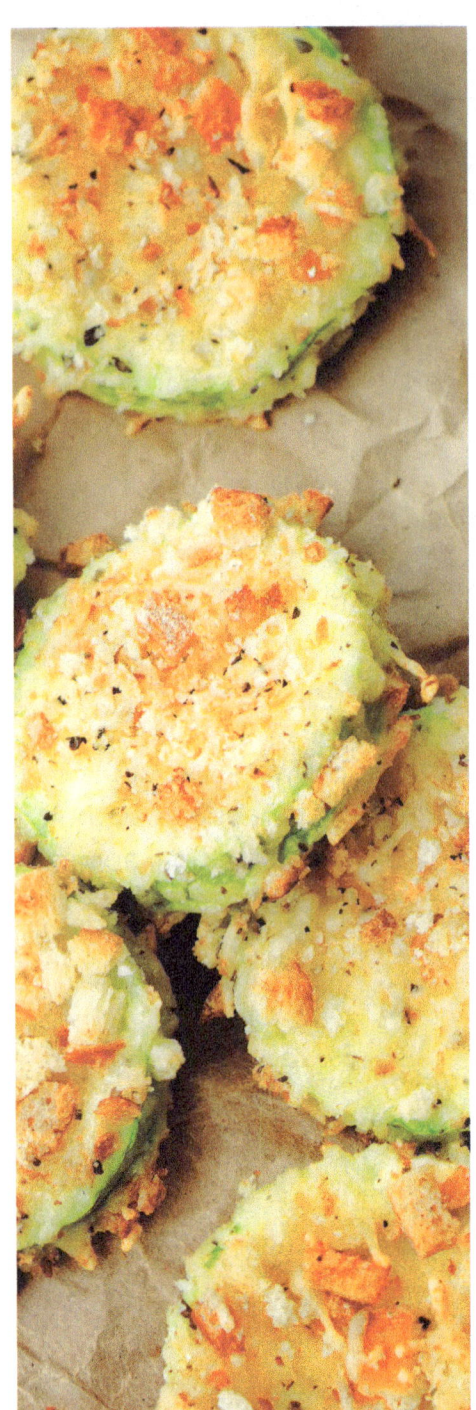

PARMESAN ZUCCHINI CHIPS

Ingredients:
- 1 large zucchini, cut into thin slices
- 1/4 cup nutritional yeast flakes
- 1 teaspoon garlic powder
- 1 teaspoon onion powder
- 2 tablespoons grated parmesan cheese

Instructions:
1. Preheat oven to 375 degrees F.
2. Line a baking sheet with parchment paper and place zucchini slices on the surface.
3. In a small bowl, mix together nutritional yeast flakes, garlic powder, onion powder, and parmesan cheese. Sprinkle over zucchini chips and bake for 20-25 minutes, or until chips are crisp. Serve immediately!

Serving Size: 1/4 cup
Calories: 130

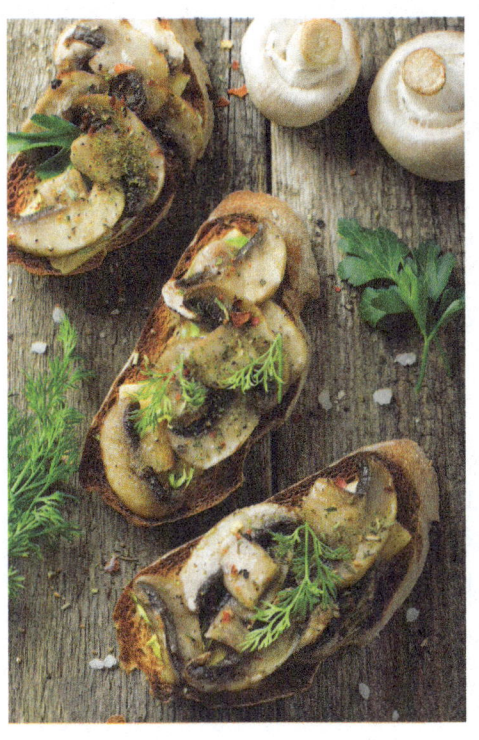

MUSHROOM CROSTINI WITH HERBS AND GARLIC

Ingredients:
- 8-10 large mushrooms, sliced
- 1/4 cup olive oil
- 3 cloves garlic, minced
- 1 tablespoon chopped fresh parsley
- 1 tablespoon chopped fresh thyme
- Salt and pepper to taste

For the crostini:
- 1 baguette, cut into 1/2-inch slices

Instructions:
1. Preheat oven to 375 degrees F.
2. In a large bowl, mix together mushrooms, olive oil, garlic, parsley, thyme, salt and pepper.
3. Place mushroom mixture on a baking sheet and bake for 20-25 minutes, or until mushrooms are cooked through.
4. Meanwhile, toast baguette slices in the oven for 5-7 minutes, or until golden brown.
5. To assemble, top each baguette slice with a few cooked mushrooms and serve immediately!

Serving Size: 1 crostini
Calories: 110

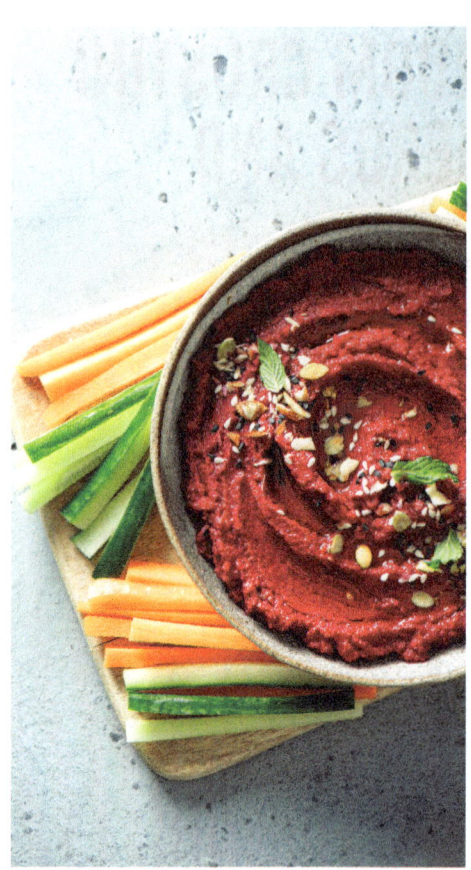

ROASTED BEET HUMMUS WITH CARROT STICKS

Ingredients:
- 2 large beets, peeled and diced
- 1 15-ounce can chickpeas, drained and rinsed
- 1/4 cup tahini
- 3 cloves garlic, minced
- 1/4 cup freshly squeezed lemon juice
- 1 teaspoon ground cumin
- Salt and pepper to taste

For the carrot sticks:
- 1 pound carrots, peeled and cut into 3-inch sticks

Instructions:
1. Preheat oven to 375 degrees F.
2. Line a baking sheet with parchment paper and place beet cubes on the surface. Bake for 25-30 minutes, or until beets are cooked through.
3. In a food processor, combine cooked beets, chickpeas, tahini, garlic, lemon juice, cumin, salt and pepper. Blend until smooth.
4. Serve beet hummus with carrot sticks and enjoy!

Serving Size: 1/4 cup
Calories: 90

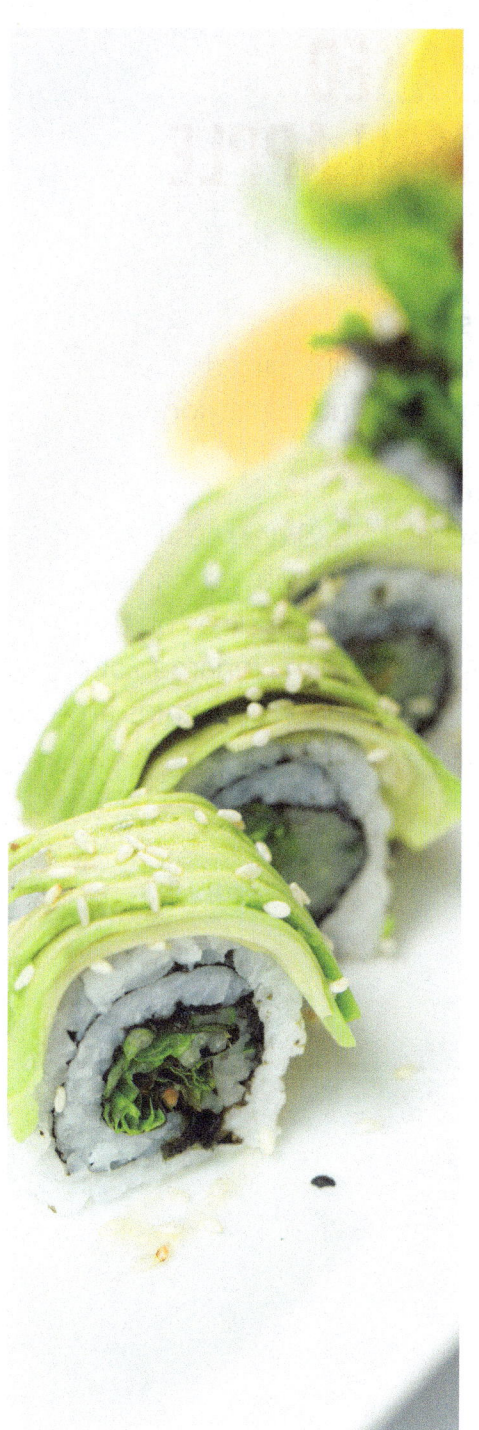

CUCUMBER AVOCADO SUSHI ROLLS

Ingredients:
- 1 large cucumber, peeled and cut into thin strips
- 1 avocado, diced
- 1/4 cup cooked brown rice
- 2 tablespoons finely chopped nori seaweed sheets

Instructions:
1. In a medium bowl, mix together cucumber strips, avocado, brown rice, and nori seaweed.
2. To assemble sushi rolls, take one strip of cucumber and place it on a flat surface. Top with a spoonful of avocado mixture and roll up tightly. Repeat until all cucumber strips are used up. Serve immediately!

Serving Size: 1 sushi roll
Calories: 120

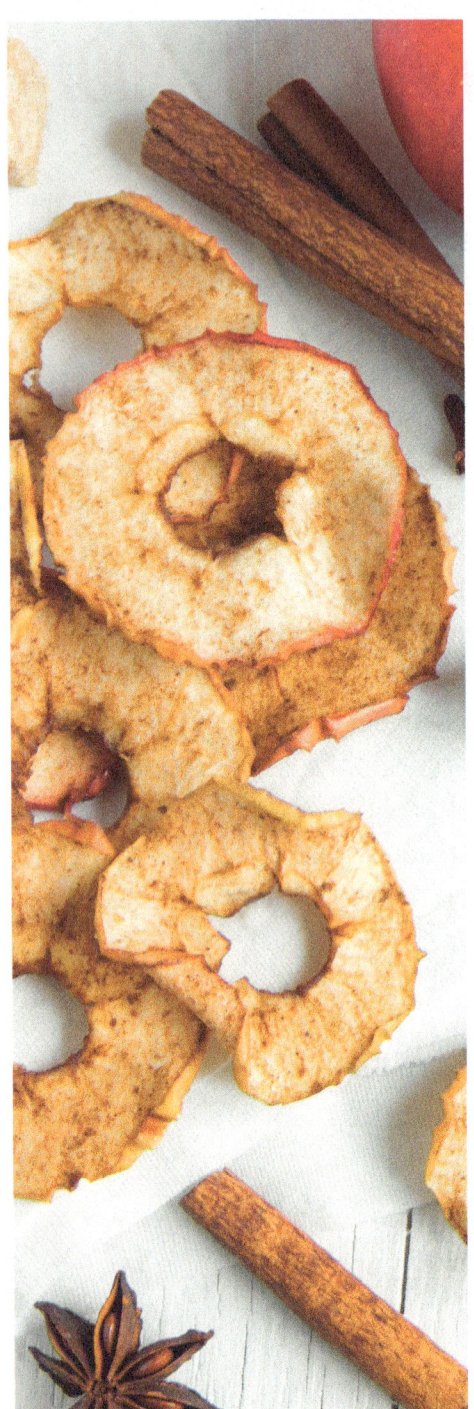

OVEN BAKED CINNAMON APPLE CHIPS

Ingredients:
- 2 large apples, thinly sliced
- 1 teaspoon ground cinnamon

Instructions:
1. Preheat oven to 225 degrees F.
2. Line a baking sheet with parchment paper and place apple slices on the surface. Sprinkle with cinnamon and bake for 1-2 hours, or until chips are crisp. Enjoy!

Serving Size: 1/4 cup
Calories: 80

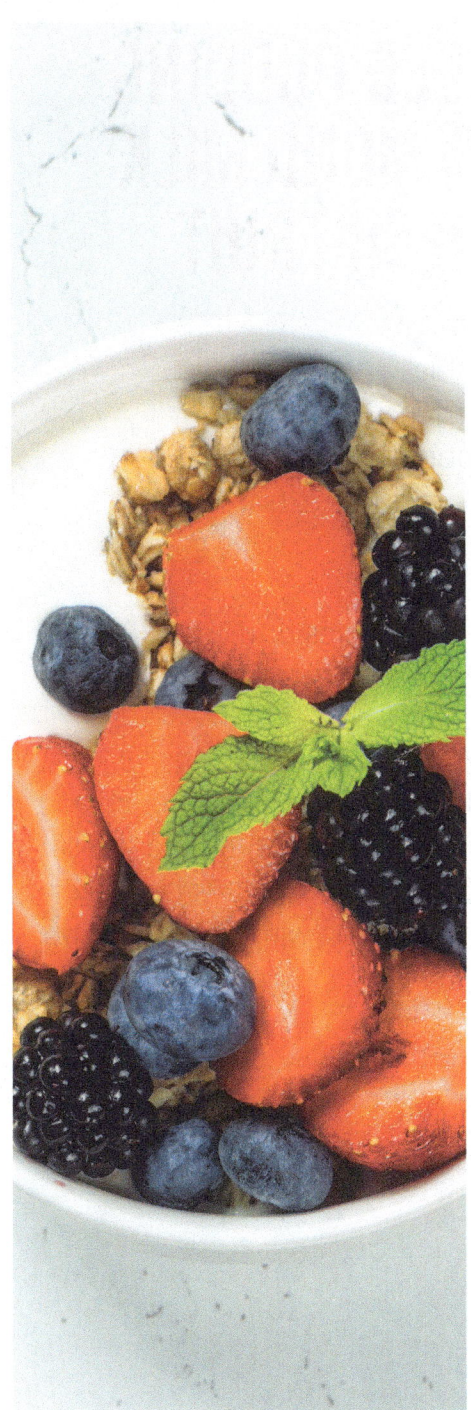

GREEK YOGURT WITH HONEY AND BERRIES

Ingredients:
- 1 cup plain Greek yogurt
- 1/4 cup honey
- 1 cup mixed berries

Instructions:
1. In a medium bowl, mix together yogurt, honey, and berries. Serve immediately!

Serving Size: 1 cup
Calories: 190

CHIA SEED PUDDING WITH ALMOND MILK AND FRESH FRUIT

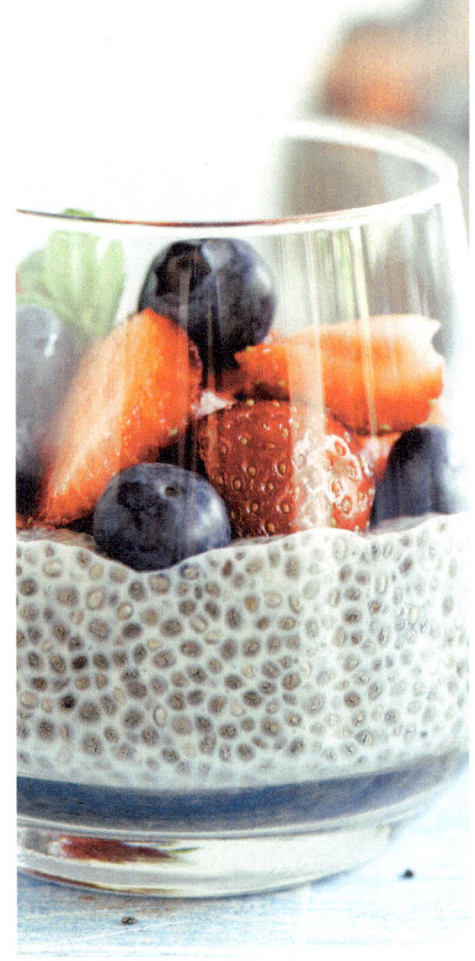

Ingredients:
- 1/4 cup chia seeds
- 1 cup almond milk
- 2 tablespoons honey
- 1 teaspoon vanilla extract

For the fresh fruit:
- 1 cup mixed berries or diced fruit of choice

Instructions:
1. In a medium bowl, mix together chia seeds, almond milk, honey, and vanilla extract. Let sit for 5 minutes to thicken.
2. Serve chia pudding with fresh fruit and enjoy!

Serving Size: 1 cup
Calories: 210

CHAPTER THREE:
Breakfasts

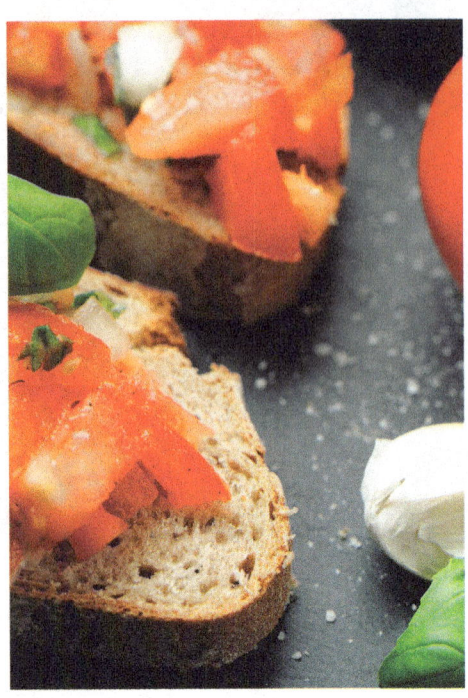

SMASHED CHICKPEA BRUSCHETTA

Ingredients:
- 1 can (15 oz) chickpeas, drained and rinsed
- 1/2 cup of sliced tomatoes (optional sub)
- 1/4 cup diced red onion
- 1 clove garlic, minced
- 1/4 cup chopped fresh parsley
- Juice of 1/2 a lemon
- Salt (optional) and black pepper (optional) to taste
- 3 tablespoons olive oil, divided
- 1 baguette, sliced into 1-inch pieces

Instructions:
1. Preheat oven to 375 degrees F.
2. In a medium bowl, use a fork or potato masher to mash together chickpeas, red onion, garlic, parsley, lemon juice, salt and black pepper (optional).
3. Drizzle in 2 tablespoons of olive oil and mix until well combined.
4. Spread mixture onto baguette slices and drizzle with remaining olive oil.
5. Place on a baking sheet and bake for 15-20 minutes, or until bread is toasted and chickpea mixture is hot. Serve immediately!

Serving Size: 1 slice
Calories: 140

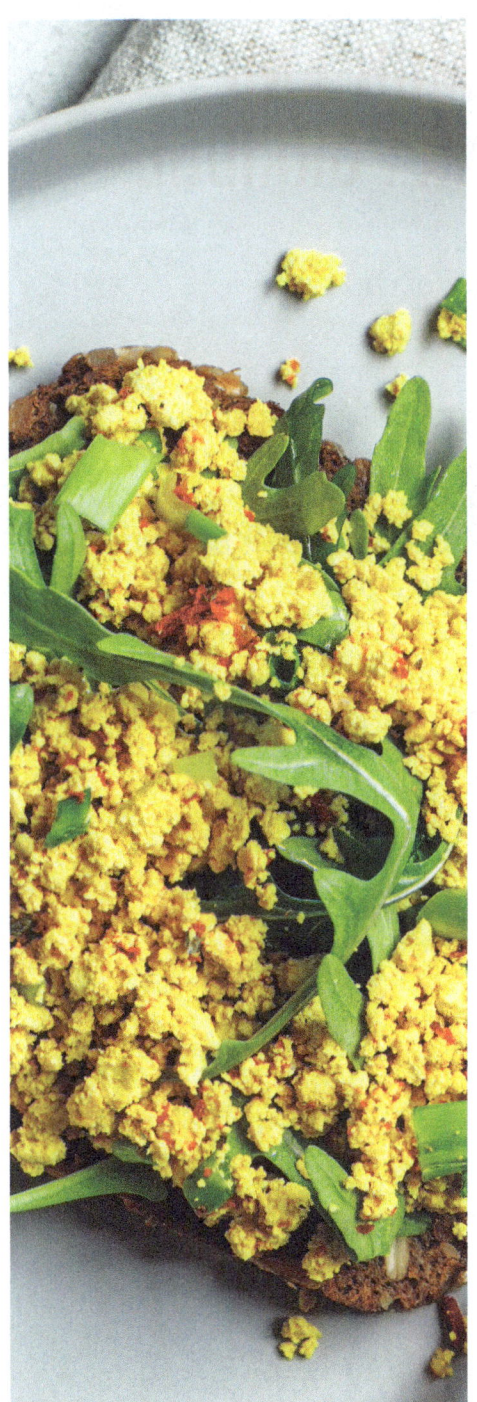

TOFU SCRAMBLE

Ingredients:

- 1 tablespoon olive oil
- 1/2 cup diced onion
- 3 cloves garlic, minced
- 1 block (14 oz) extra-firm tofu, drained and crumbled
- Turmeric, to taste
- Salt (optional) and black pepper (optional) to taste
- 1/4 cup nutritional yeast flakes

Instructions:

1. In a large skillet over medium heat, heat olive oil. Add onion and garlic and cook until both are translucent.
2. Add tofu and season with turmeric, salt and black pepper (optional) to taste. Cook for 5 minutes, or until tofu is slightly browned.
3. Stir in nutritional yeast flakes and continue to cook for 2-3 minutes, or until heated through. Serve immediately!

Serving Size: 1/2 cup
Calories: 120

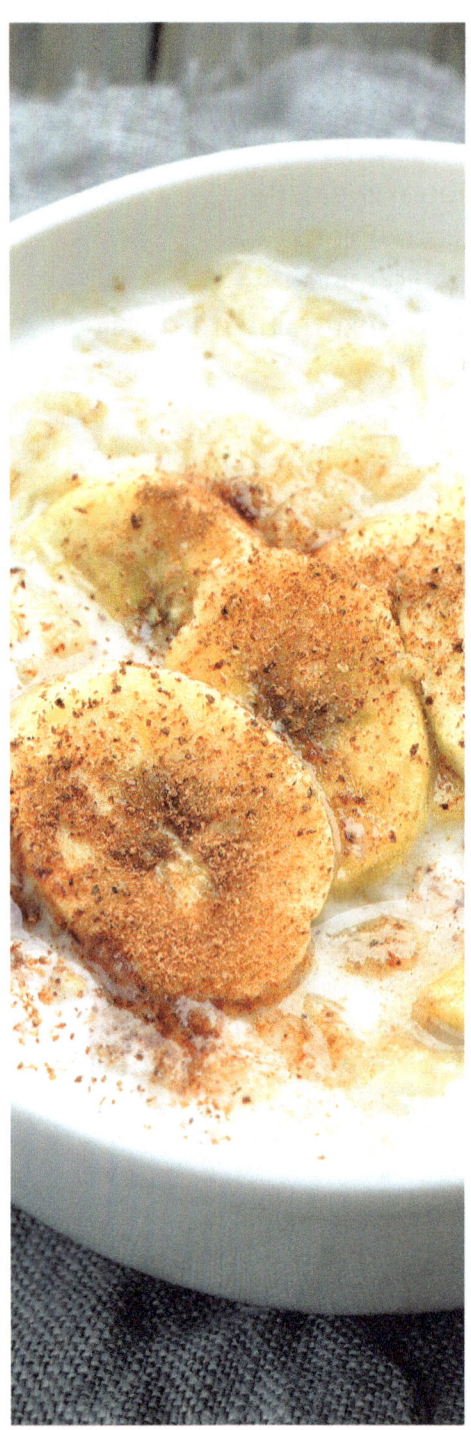

CINNAMON AND BANANA PORRIDGE

Ingredients:
- 1 cup milk of choice
- 1/2 cup rolled oats
- 1 medium banana, sliced
- 1 teaspoon ground cinnamon

Instructions:
1. In a small saucepan over medium heat, bring milk to a boil.
2. Stir in rolled oats and cook for 1 minute.
3. Remove from heat and stir in banana and cinnamon. Let sit for 2-3 minutes, or until bananas are soft. Serve immediately!

Serving Size: 1 bowl
Calories: 290

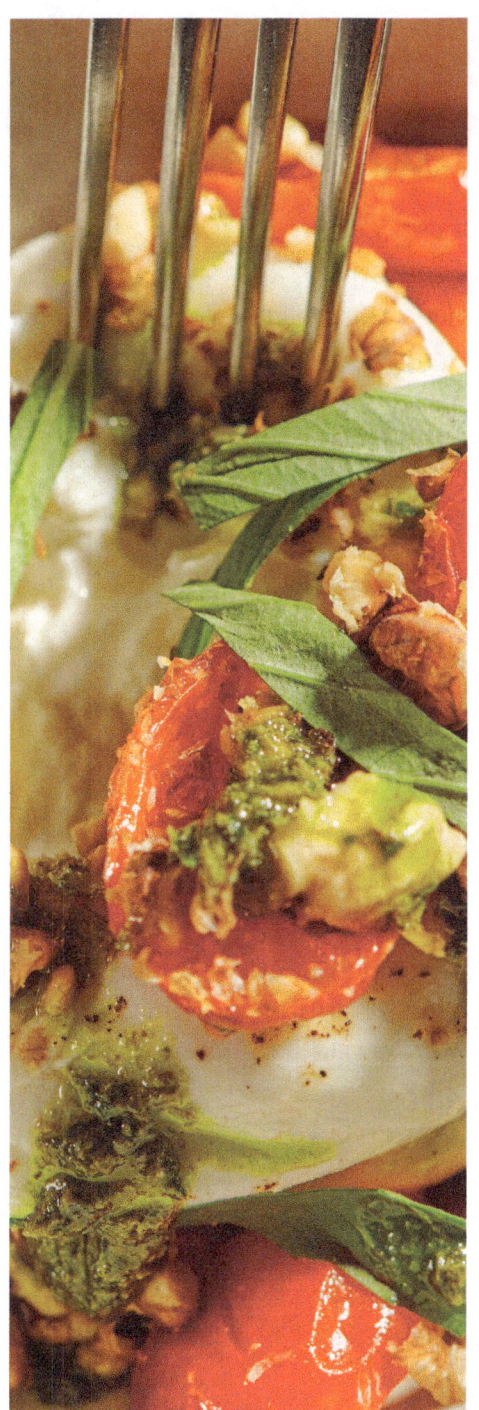

MEDITERRANEAN BREAKFAST BURRATA

Ingredients:

- 1 cup diced tomatoes
- 1/4 cup chopped fresh basil
- 1 tablespoon olive oil
- Salt (optional) and black pepper (optional) to taste
- 1 ball (8 oz) burrata cheese
- 1 baguette, sliced into 1-inch pieces

Instructions:

1. Preheat oven to 375 degrees F.
2. In a small bowl, mix together diced tomatoes, basil, olive oil, salt and black pepper (optional).
3. Cut burrata cheese into 1-inch pieces and place on top of baguette slices.
4. Top with tomato mixture and place on a baking sheet. Bake for 10-15 minutes, or until bread is toasted and cheese is hot. Serve immediately!

Serving Size: 1 slice
Calories: 210

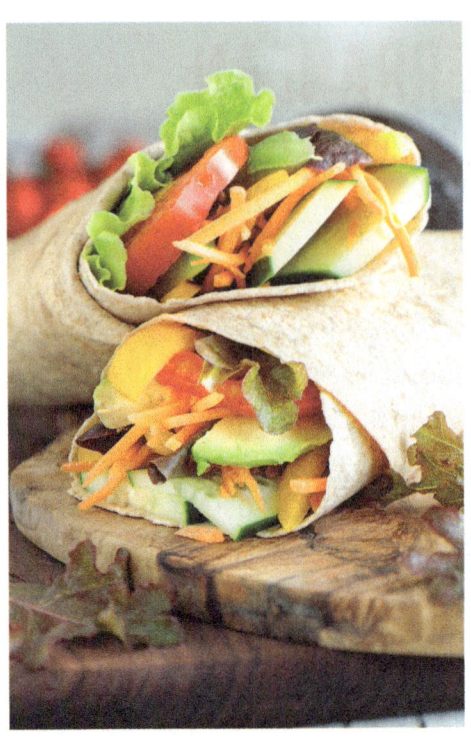

VEGAN BREAKFAST BURRITO

Ingredients:
- 1/2 cup diced onion
- 1/2 cup diced red bell pepper
- 1/2 cup diced green bell pepper
- 3 cloves garlic, minced
- 1 teaspoon ground cumin
- Salt (optional) and black pepper (optional) to taste
- 1 (15 oz) can black beans, drained and rinsed
- 6-8 eggs, scrambled (or 1/2 cup egg whites)

Instructions:
1. In a large skillet over medium heat, sauté onion, bell peppers, garlic and cumin until vegetables are soft. Season with salt and black pepper (optional) to taste.
2. Stir in black beans and cook for 2-3 minutes, or until heated through.
3. Add scrambled eggs (or egg whites) and cook for 5 minutes, or until eggs are firm.
4. 4Serve mixture on whole wheat tortillas and enjoy!

Serving Size: 1 burrito
Calories: 340

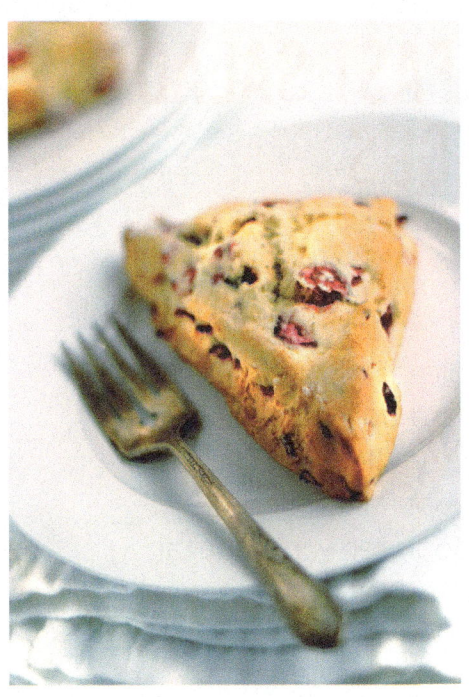

LOW-SUGAR CRANBERRY ORANGE SCONES

Ingredients:
- 2 cups whole wheat flour
- 1 tablespoon baking powder
- 1/4 teaspoon salt
- 6 tablespoons cold vegan butter
- 1/2 cup + 2 tablespoons non-dairy milk
- 1/2 cup fresh or frozen cranberries
- 1/4 cup cane sugar
- 1 teaspoon orange zest

Instructions:
1. Preheat oven to 400 degrees F.
2. In a large bowl, whisk together whole wheat flour, baking powder and salt. Cut in vegan butter until mixture resembles coarse crumbs.
3. Stir in non-dairy milk, cranberries, sugar and orange zest until dough comes together.
4. Place dough on a lightly floured surface and knead for 10-12 times. Pat into a 1-inch thick circle and use a biscuit cutter to cut out 8 scones.
5. Place on a baking sheet and bake for 12-14 minutes, or until scones are golden brown. Serve immediately!

Serving Size: 1 scone
Calories: 210

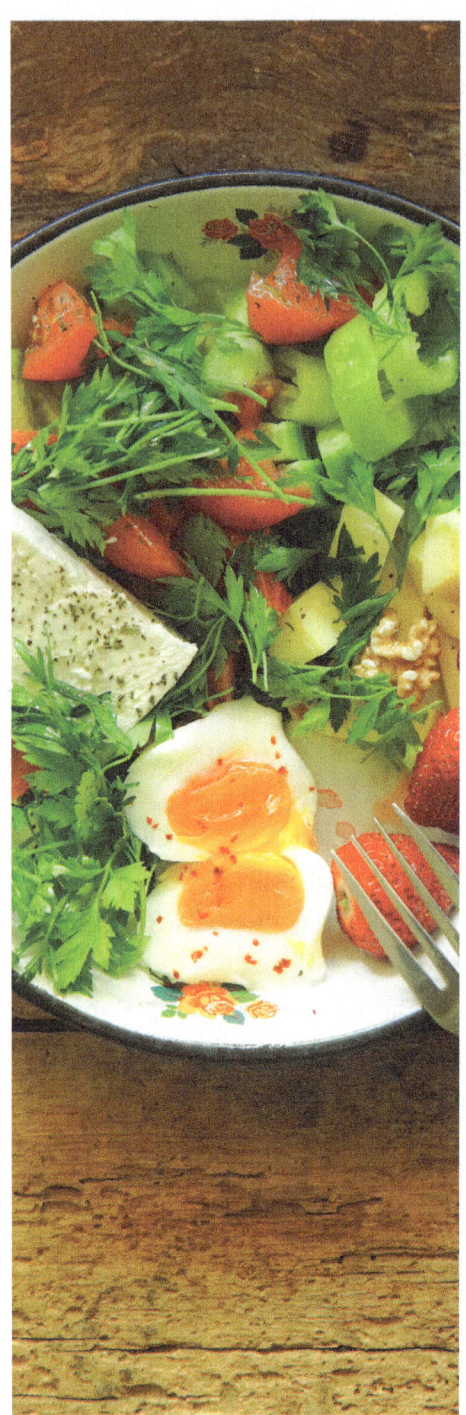

BREAKFAST SALAD WITH EGGS

Ingredients:

- 1 head Romaine lettuce, chopped
- 1/2 cup diced tomatoes
- 1/4 cup diced red onion
- 3 eggs, hard-boiled and chopped
- 1/4 cup crumbled feta cheese
- 1 tablespoon olive oil
- 1 tablespoon red wine vinegar
- Salt (optional) and black pepper (optional) to taste

Instructions:

1. In a large bowl, mix together Romaine lettuce, tomatoes, red onion and eggs.
2. Top with feta cheese, olive oil and red wine vinegar. Season with salt and black pepper (optional) to taste. Serve immediately!

Serving Size: 1 salad
Calories: 190

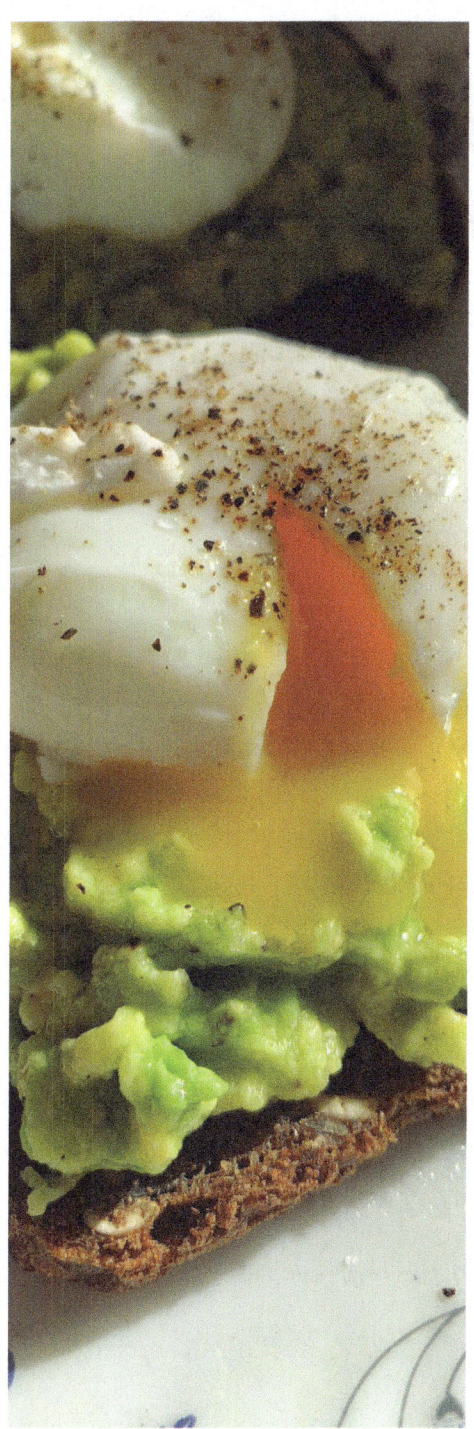

AVOCADO TOAST WITH EGG

Ingredients:
- 2 slices whole wheat bread, toasted
- 1/2 avocado, mashed
- 1 egg, fried or scrambled
- Salt (optional) and black pepper (optional) to taste

Instructions:
1. Spread avocado on toast and top with egg. Season with salt and black pepper (optional) to taste. Serve immediately!

Serving Size: 1 toast
Calories: 290

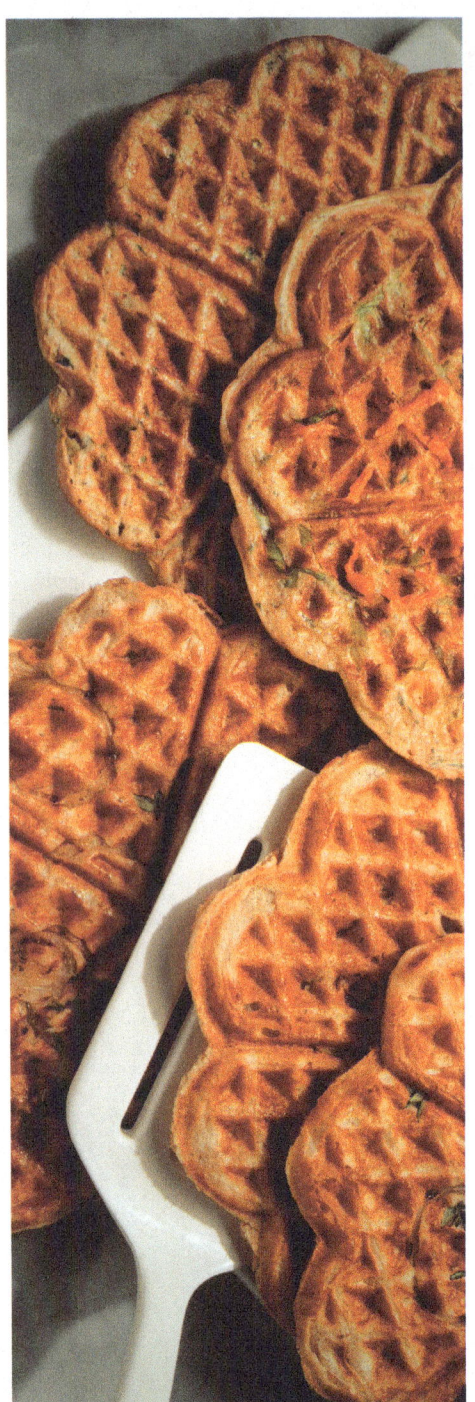

SPICY WAFFLED CAULIFLOWER HASH BROWNS

Ingredients:
- 1/2 head cauliflower, grated
- 1/4 cup diced onion
- 1 clove garlic, minced
- 1/4 teaspoon cumin
- 1/4 teaspoon chili powder
- Salt (optional) and black pepper (optional) to taste

Instructions:
1. Preheat waffle iron to medium-high heat.
2. In a large bowl, mix together cauliflower, onion, garlic, cumin, chili powder, salt and black pepper (optional).
3. Place 1/4 of the mixture on the waffle iron and cook for 3-5 minutes, or until golden brown and crispy. Repeat with remaining cauliflower mixture. Serve immediately!

Serving Size: 1 hash brown
Calories: 30

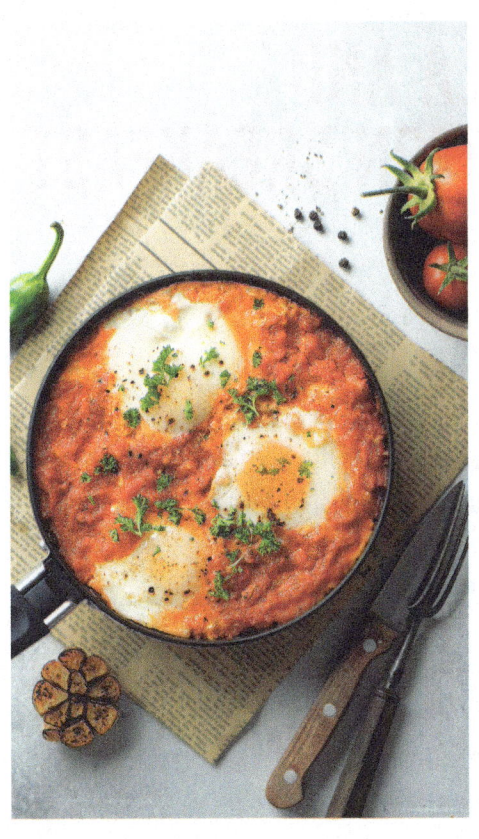

SWEET POTATO, BEAN, AND KALE SHAKSHUKA

Ingredients:
- 1 tablespoon olive oil
- 1 small sweet potato, peeled and diced
- 1/2 cup diced onion
- 3 cloves garlic, minced
- 1 teaspoon ground cumin
- alt (optional) and black pepper (optional) to taste
- 1 (15 oz) can diced tomatoes, undrained
- 1/4 cup tomato paste
- 1 (15 oz) can black beans, drained and rinsed
- 1 bunch kale, stems removed and leaves chopped

Instructions:
1. In a large skillet over medium heat, sauté sweet potato, onion, garlic and cumin in olive oil until vegetables are soft. Season with salt and black pepper (optional) to taste.
2. Stir in diced tomatoes, tomato paste, black beans and kale. Bring to a simmer and cook for 10 minutes, or until kale is wilted.
3. Serve shakshuka immediately with whole wheat bread or pita bread!

Serving Size: 1/6 of recipe
Calories: 190

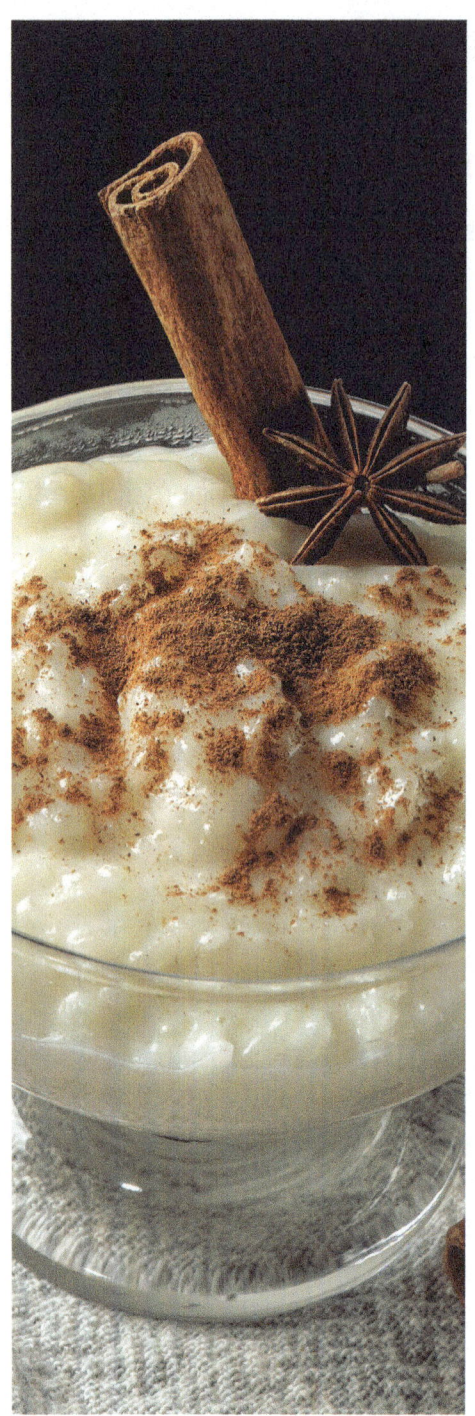

VANILLA AND CINNAMON BREAKFAST RICE

Ingredients:
- 1 cup cooked rice
- 1/2 cup non-dairy milk
- 1/4 teaspoon vanilla extract
- 1/4 teaspoon ground cinnamon

Instructions:
1. In a small pot over low heat, cook rice in non-dairy milk until hot and creamy.
2. Stir in vanilla extract and cinnamon. Serve immediately!

Serving Size: 1/2 recipe
Calories: 200

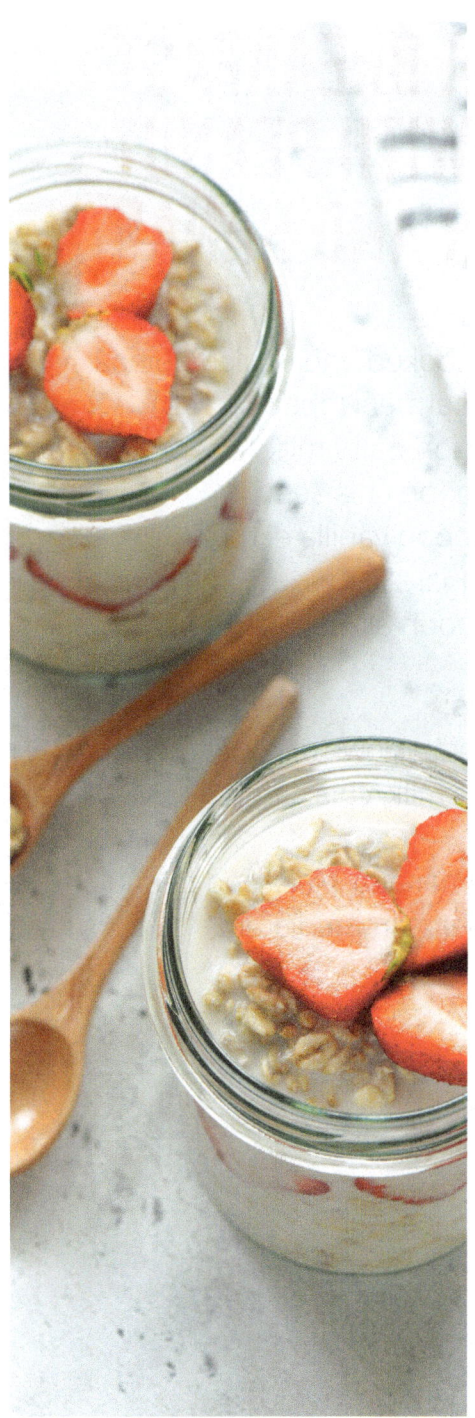

OVERNIGHT OATS WITH STRAWBERRY AND PASSIONFRUIT

Ingredients:
- 1/2 cup rolled oats
- 1/2 cup non-dairy milk
- 1/4 cup diced strawberries
- 1 tablespoon chia seeds
- 1/4 teaspoon vanilla extract
- Pinch of ground cinnamon

Instructions:
1. In a medium bowl, mix together all ingredients. Cover and refrigerate overnight.
2. In the morning, stir oats and add more non-dairy milk if desired. Top with additional diced strawberries and passionfruit (optional). Serve immediately!

Serving Size: 1/2 recipe
Calories: 220

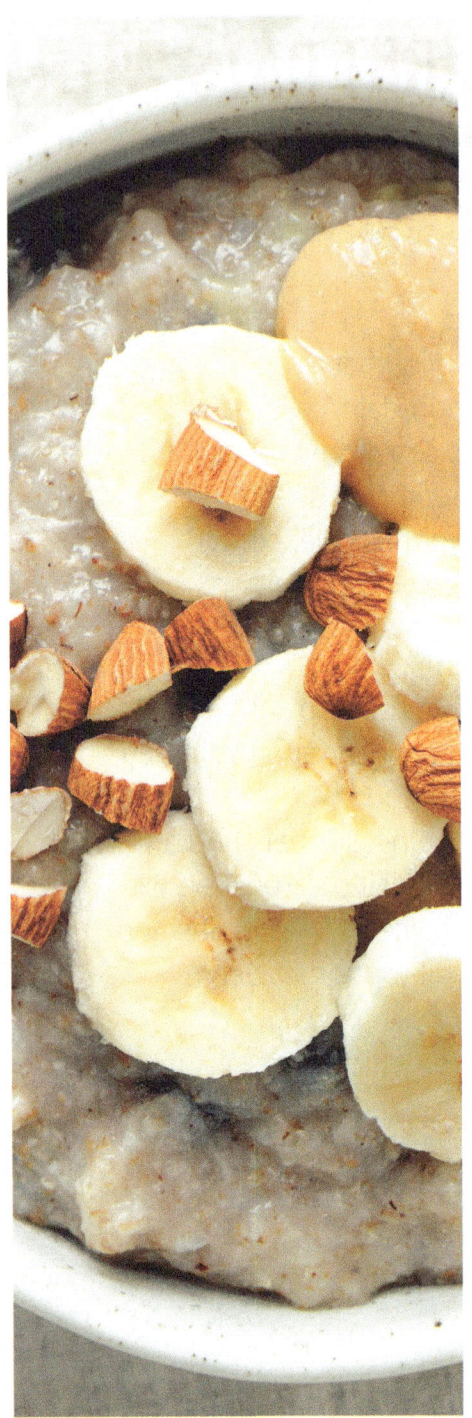

QUINOA BREAKFAST BOWL WITH PEANUT BUTTER AND BANANA

Ingredients:
- 1/2 cup cooked and cooled quinoa
- 1/2 cup oatmeal (optional sub)
- 1/2 cup non-dairy milk
- 1 tablespoon chia seeds
- 1/2 teaspoon vanilla extract
- 1/2 banana, sliced
- 1 tablespoon all-natural peanut butter

Instructions:
1. In a medium bowl, mix together quinoa, non-dairy milk, chia seeds and vanilla extract.
2. Top with banana slices and peanut butter. Serve immediately!

Serving Size: 1 bowl
Calories: 290

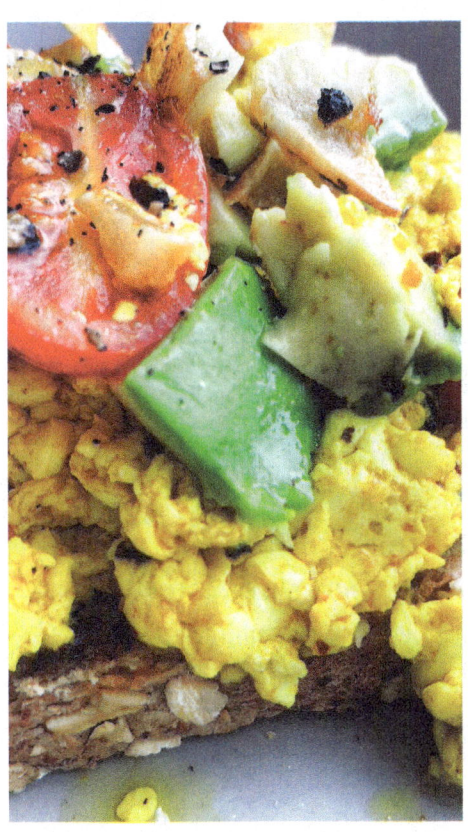

CHICKPEA SCRAMBLE WITH TOMATO AND AVOCADO

Ingredients:
- 1 tablespoon olive oil
- 1/4 cup diced onion
- 3 cloves garlic, minced
- 1 (15 oz) can chickpeas, drained and rinsed
- 1/4 teaspoon ground turmeric
- 1/4 teaspoon chili powder
- Salt (optional) and black pepper (optional) to taste
- 1/2 cup diced tomatoes
- 1/2 avocado, diced

Instructions:
1. In a large skillet over medium heat, sauté onion and garlic in olive oil until softened.
2. Stir in chickpeas and season with turmeric, chili powder, salt and black pepper (optional). Cook for 5 minutes.
3. Add diced tomatoes and cook for an additional 3 minutes. Remove from heat and stir in avocado. Serve immediately!

Serving Size: 1/2 recipe
Calories: 280

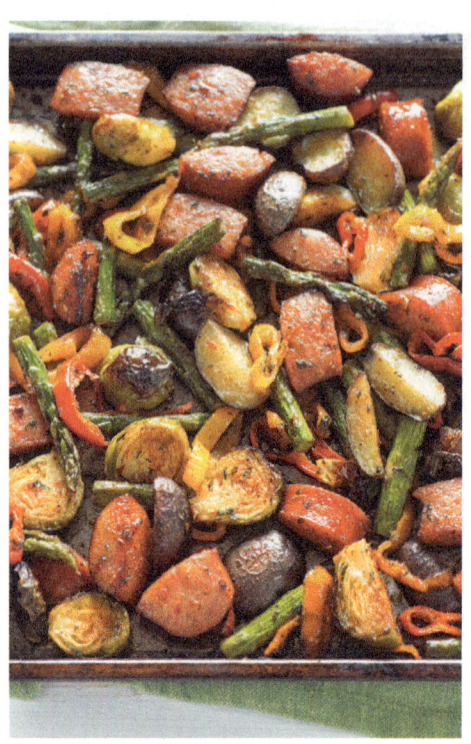

SHEET-PAN VEGAN SAUSAGE AND VEGETABLES

Ingredients:
- 1/2 teaspoon dried oregano
- 1/2 teaspoon dried thyme
- 1/4 teaspoon paprika
- Salt (optional) and black pepper (optional) to taste
- 1 lb vegan sausage, sliced into 1" pieces
- 3 cups chopped broccoli florets
- 3 cups chopped cauliflower florets
- 2 tablespoons olive oil, divided

Instructions:
1. Preheat oven to 400°F. Line a baking sheet with parchment paper.
2. In a small bowl, mix together oregano, thyme, paprika, salt and black pepper (optional). Set aside.
3. In a large bowl, mix together vegan sausage, broccoli and cauliflower. Drizzle with 1 tablespoon olive oil and toss to coat.
4. Spread mixture onto the prepared baking sheet. Bake for 20 minutes, or until vegetables are tender and sausage is browned. Remove from oven and serve immediately!

Serving Size: 1/6 of recipe
Calories: 220

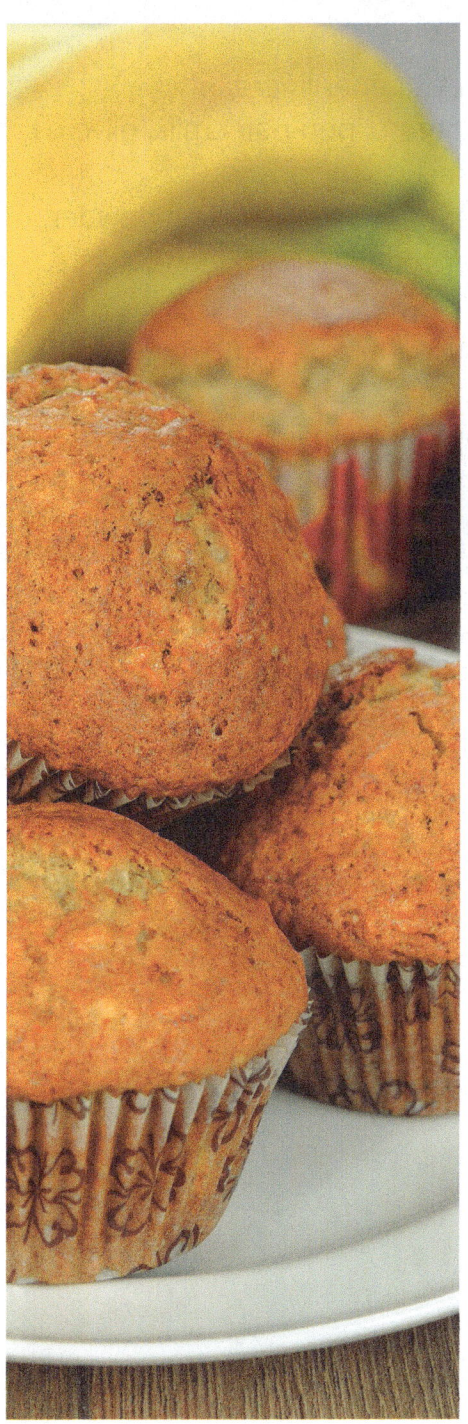

SWEET POTATO BANANA MUFFINS

Ingredients:

- 1 cup mashed sweet potato
- 1/2 cup non-dairy milk
- 1/4 cup olive oil
- 1/4 cup agave nectar or maple syrup
- 2 teaspoons vanilla extract
- 1 1/2 cups whole wheat pastry flour
- 1 teaspoon baking powder
- 1 teaspoon baking soda
- 1/2 teaspoon ground cinnamon
- Pinch of ground nutmeg (optional)
- Salt (optional) to taste
- 1/2 cup diced banana, divided

Instructions:

1. Preheat oven to 350°F. Line a muffin tin with 12 paper liners.
2. In a large bowl, mix together mashed sweet potato, non-dairy milk, olive oil, agave nectar or maple syrup, and vanilla extract.
3. In a separate bowl, mix together whole wheat pastry flour, baking powder, baking soda, cinnamon and nutmeg (optional). Add salt (optional) to taste. Stir until well combined.
4. Add dry ingredients to wet ingredients and mix until just combined. Gently fold in 1/4 cup banana diced.
5. Divide batter evenly among muffin liners. Top with remaining 1/4 cup banana diced. Bake for 18-20 minutes, or until a toothpick inserted into the center of a muffin comes out clean. Remove from oven and let cool for 5 minutes before serving. Enjoy!

Serving Size: 1 muffin
Calories: 190

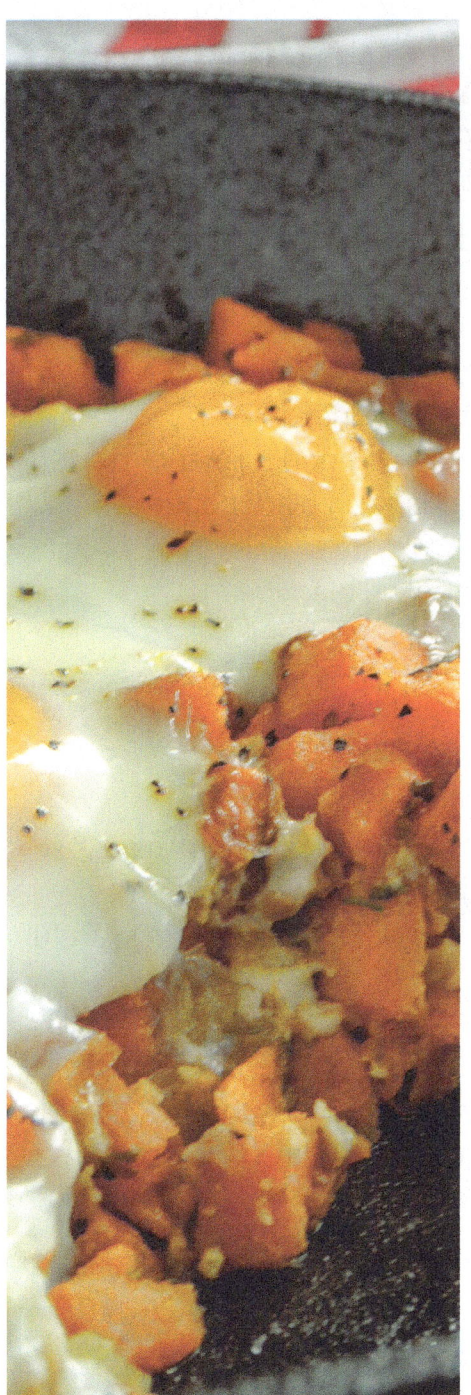

BUTTERNUT SQUASH HASH WITH FRIED EGGS

Ingredients:
- 1 tablespoon olive oil
- 1/2 cup diced onion
- 3 cloves garlic, minced
- 2 cups peeled and diced butternut squash
- Salt (optional) and black pepper (optional) to taste
- 4 large eggs

Instructions:
1. In a large skillet over medium heat, sauté onion and garlic in olive oil until softened.
2. Stir in butternut squash and season with salt and black pepper (optional). Cook for 10 minutes, or until squash is tender.
3. Using a spoon, make 4 indentations in the hash. Crack an egg into each indentation. Cover pan and cook for 5-7 minutes, or until eggs are cooked to your liking. Remove from heat and serve immediately!

Serving Size: 1/4 of recipe
Calories: 220

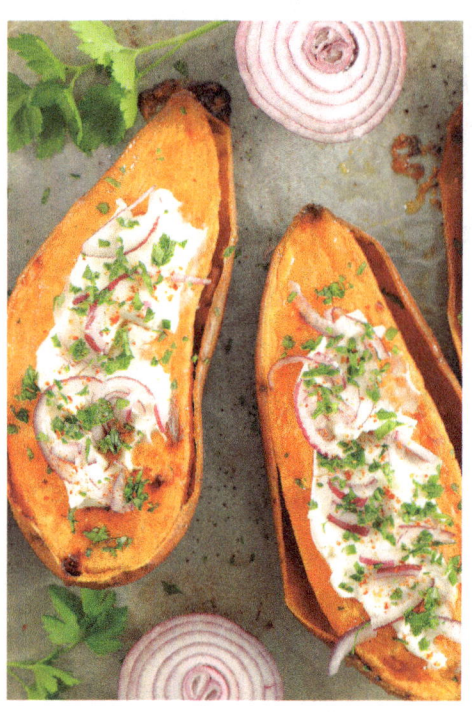

BREAKFAST LOADED SWEET POTATO

Ingredients:

- 1 large sweet potato, baked
- 1/4 cup non-dairy milk
- 2 tablespoons finely diced onion
- 1 clove garlic, minced
- 1/4 teaspoon ground turmeric
- Salt (optional) and black pepper (optional) to taste
- 1/4 cup cooked black beans
- 2 tablespoons salsa
- 1/4 avocado, diced

Instructions:

1. Preheat oven to 350°F.
2. In a small bowl, mix together non-dairy milk, onion, garlic and turmeric. Season with salt and black pepper (optional). Set aside.
3. Cut a sweet potato in half lengthwise and scoop out the flesh, being careful not to break the skin.
4. In a medium bowl, mash the sweet potato flesh with a fork. Mix in the milk mixture until well combined.
5. Spoon the sweet potato mixture back into the skins. Top with black beans, salsa and avocado. Bake for 10-15 minutes, or until heated through. Serve immediately!

Serving Size: 1/2 of recipe
Calories: 290

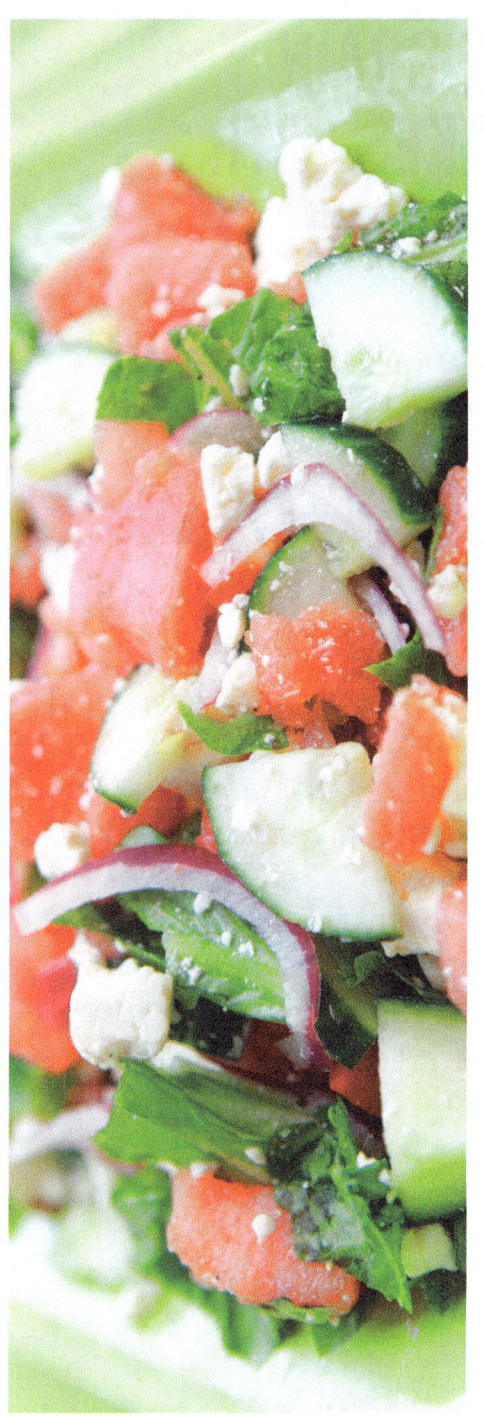

WATERMELON AND BERRY SALAD WITH BUCKWHEAT

Ingredients:

- 1 cup cubed watermelon
- 1 cup mixed berries (strawberries, blueberries, raspberries, etc.)
- 1/4 cup finely diced red onion
- 2 tablespoons chopped fresh mint leaves
- 2 tablespoons balsamic vinegar
- 1 tablespoon olive oil
- Salt (optional) and black pepper (optional) to taste
- 1/4 cup cooked buckwheat groats

Instructions:

1. In a large bowl, mix together watermelon, berries, red onion and mint leaves.
2. In a small bowl, whisk together balsamic vinegar, olive oil and salt and black pepper (optional). Pour over the salad and mix until well coated.
3. 3Gently stir in buckwheat groats. Serve immediately or refrigerate for later!

Serving Size: 1/4 of recipe
Calories: 150

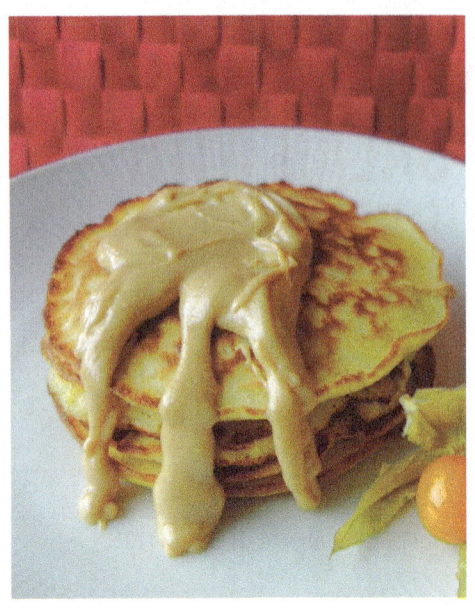

WHOLE GRAIN PANCAKES WITH CASHEW BUTTER

Ingredients:
- 1 cup whole wheat pastry flour
- 1 tablespoon baking powder
- 1/4 teaspoon salt (optional)
- 1 cup non-dairy milk
- 1 tablespoon olive oil or melted non-dairy butter, plus more for cooking

Instructions:
1. In a large bowl, mix together whole wheat pastry flour, baking powder and salt (optional).
2. In a small bowl, whisk together non-dairy milk and olive oil or melted non-dairy butter. Pour into the dry ingredients and mix until just combined. Do not overmix!
3. Heat a large skillet over medium heat and coat with olive oil or non-dairy butter. Scoop 1/4 cup batter onto the skillet for each pancake. Cook for 2-3 minutes, or until bubbles form and the edges look dry. Flip and cook for an additional 1-2 minutes, or until golden brown. Serve immediately with cashew butter, syrup or your favorite toppings!

Serving Size: 4 pancakes
Calories: 320

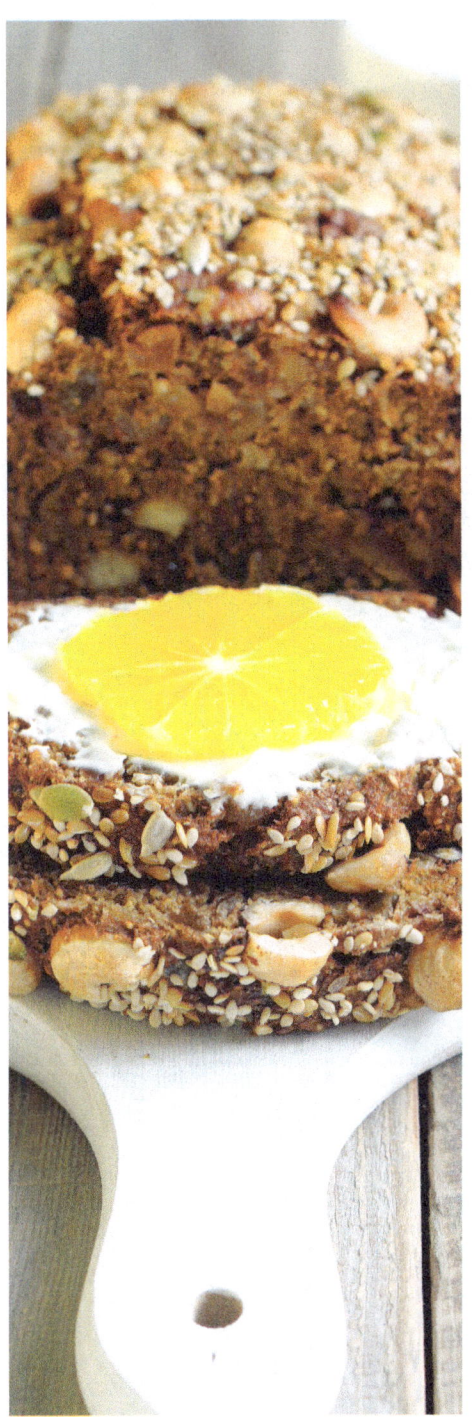

FIG, NUT, AND SEED BREAD WITH RICOTTA AND FRUIT

Ingredients:
- 1 cup whole wheat flour
- 1 cup almond meal
- 2 tablespoons flaxseed meal
- 2 teaspoons baking powder
- 1/4 teaspoon salt (optional)
- 1/2 teaspoon ground cinnamon
- 1 cup non-dairy milk
- 1/4 cup honey or agave nectar
- 1 tablespoon olive oil or melted non-dairy butter
- 1 teaspoon vanilla extract
- 6 figs, diced
- 1/4 cup chopped nuts (almonds, pecans, etc.)
- 2 tablespoons seeds (sunflower, pumpkin, etc.)

Instructions:

1. Preheat oven to 350°F. Grease a loaf pan with olive oil or non-dairy butter and set aside.
2. In a large bowl, mix together whole wheat flour, almond meal, flaxseed meal, baking powder, salt (optional) and cinnamon.
3. In a small bowl, whisk together non-dairy milk, honey or agave nectar, olive oil or melted non-dairy butter and vanilla extract. Pour into the dry ingredients and mix until just combined. Do not overmix! Fold in figs, nuts and seeds.
4. Pour batter into the prepared loaf pan and bake for 45-55 minutes, or until a toothpick inserted into the center comes out clean. Allow to cool for 10 minutes before slicing and serving. Enjoy!

Serving Size: 1 slice
Calories: 210

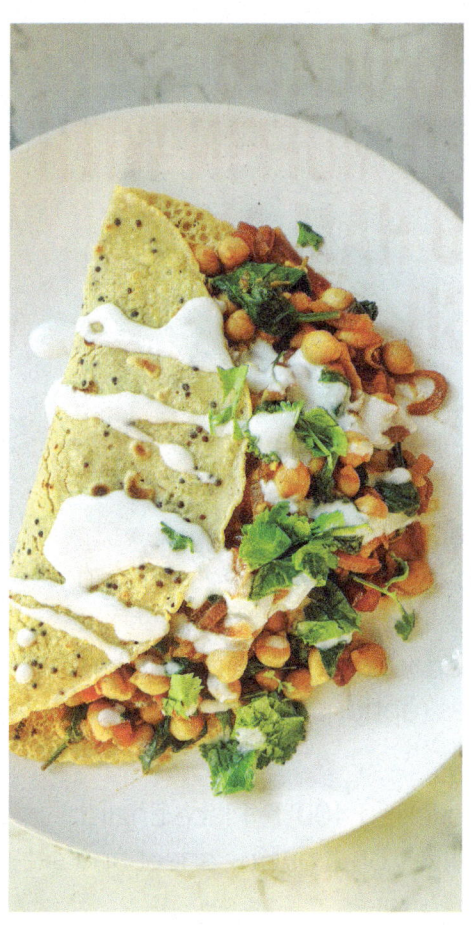

CURRIED CHICKPEA SALAD WRAPS

Ingredients:

- 1 can (15 oz) chickpeas, drained and rinsed
- 1/4 cup diced red onion
- 1/4 cup diced celery
- 1/4 cup diced green apple
- 2 tablespoons chopped fresh cilantro leaves
- 2 tablespoons raisins (optional)
- 1 tablespoon olive oil or non-dairy yogurt
- 1 tablespoon freshly squeezed lemon juice
- 1 teaspoon curry powder
- Salt (optional) and black pepper (optional) to taste

Instructions:

1. In a large bowl, mix together chickpeas, red onion, celery, green apple and cilantro leaves.
2. In a small bowl, whisk together raisins (optional), olive oil or non-dairy yogurt, lemon juice and curry powder. Pour over the salad and mix until well coated. Season with salt and black pepper (optional) to taste.
3. Serve immediately or refrigerate for later! Enjoy as is, or serve in a whole grain wrap with your favorite toppings.

Serving Size: 1/4 of recipe
Calories: 190

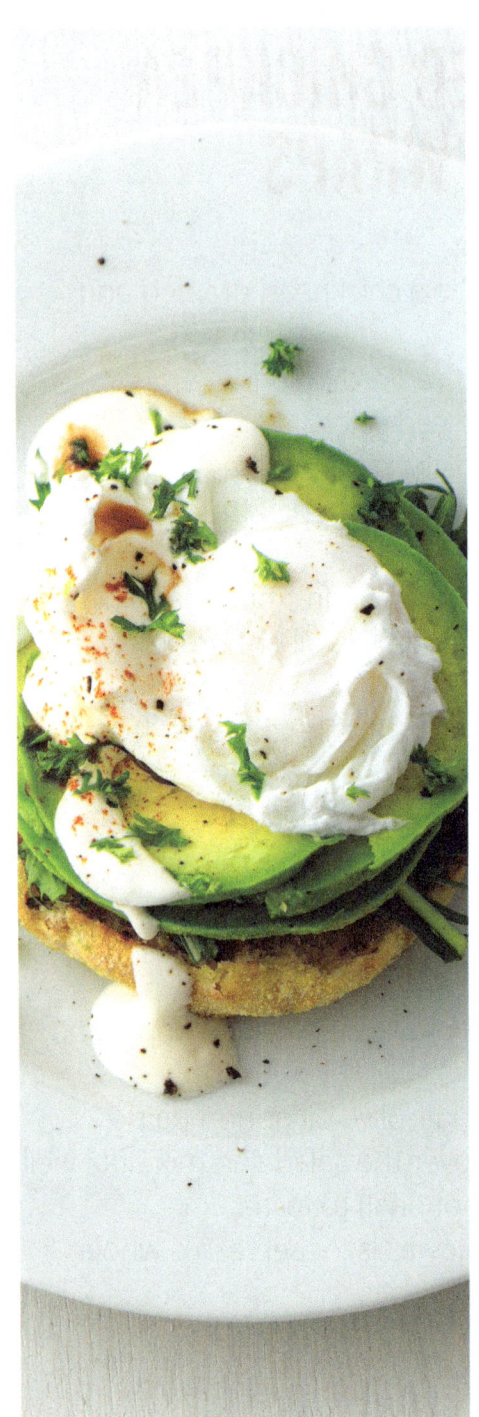

SPICY AVOCADO TOASTED MUFFIN WITH SHAVED HAM AND SPINACH

Ingredients:
- 1 whole wheat English muffin, split in half
- 1/2 avocado, diced
- 1 slice sharp cheddar cheese, shredded
- 1 slice cooked ham, shaved
- 1-2 tablespoons fresh spinach leaves
- Chili flakes (optional) to taste

Instructions:
1. Preheat oven to 400°F. Place English muffin halves on a baking sheet and set aside.
2. In a small bowl, mix together avocado and chili flakes (optional). Spread over the top of each English muffin half. Top with shredded cheddar cheese and shaved ham.
3. Bake for 10-12 minutes, or until cheese is melted and bubbly. Remove from oven and top with fresh spinach leaves. Serve immediately!

Serving Size: 1 muffin half
Calories: 290

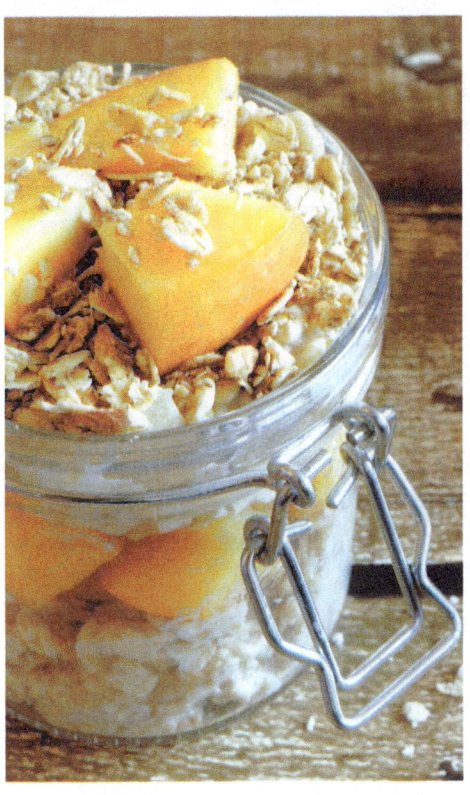

CRUNCHY OAT CLUSTERS WITH PEACH AND YOGURT

Ingredients:
- 1 cup rolled oats
- 1/4 cup sliced almonds
- 1/4 cup chopped pecans
- 1/4 cup pumpkin seeds
- 2 tablespoons chia seeds
- 1 teaspoon ground cinnamon
- 1/4 teaspoon salt (optional)
- 3/4 cup non-dairy milk
- 1/2 cup frozen peach slices, thawed and diced

Instructions:
1. Preheat oven to 375°F. Line a baking sheet with parchment paper and set aside.
2. In a large bowl, mix together rolled oats, sliced almonds, pecans, pumpkin seeds, chia seeds, ground cinnamon and salt (optional). Pour in non-dairy milk and stir until well combined. Fold in diced peach slices.
3. Drop mixture by the spoonful onto the prepared baking sheet and flatten slightly. Bake for 20-25 minutes, or until golden brown. Remove from oven and let cool for 5 minutes before serving. Enjoy!

Serving Size: 1/4 cup
Calories: 210

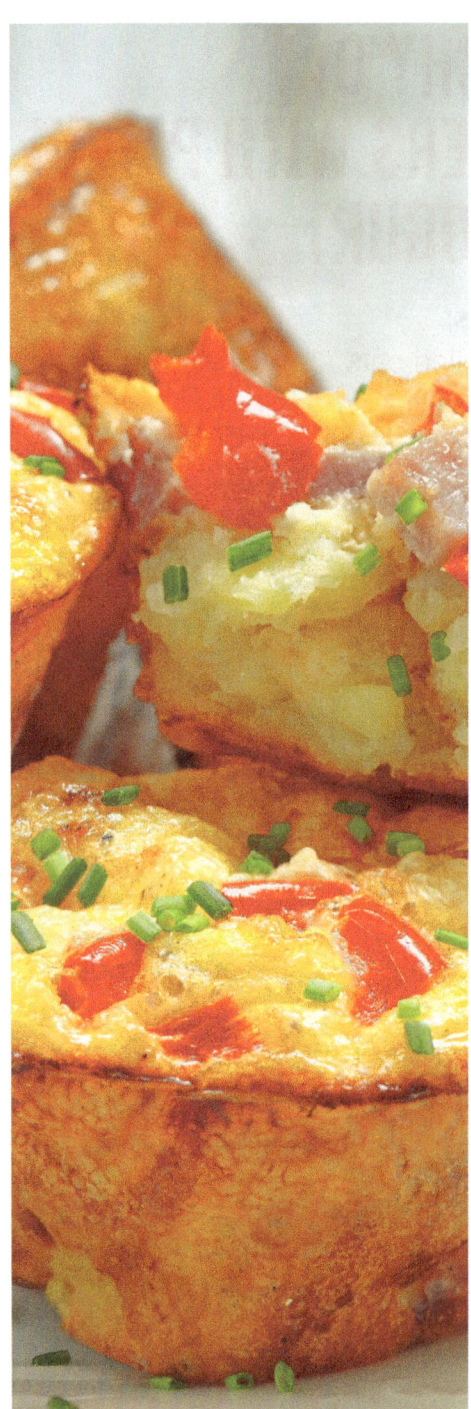

QUINOA EGG MUFFINS WITH TOMATO, BASIL AND MOZZARELLA

Ingredients:

- 1 cup cooked and cooled quinoa
- 2 large eggs, beaten
- 1/4 cup shredded mozzarella cheese
- 1/4 cup diced tomatoes
- 1 tablespoon chopped fresh basil leaves

Instructions:

1. Preheat oven to 350°F. Grease a 12-cup muffin tin with cooking spray and set aside.
2. In a large bowl, mix together cooked quinoa, eggs, mozzarella cheese, diced tomatoes and chopped basil leaves.
3. Spoon mixture evenly into the prepared muffin tin. Bake for 15-20 minutes, or until egg is firm and cooked through. Remove from oven and let cool for 5 minutes before serving. Enjoy!

Serving Size: 1 muffin
Calories: 190

CHAPTER FOUR:
Lunches

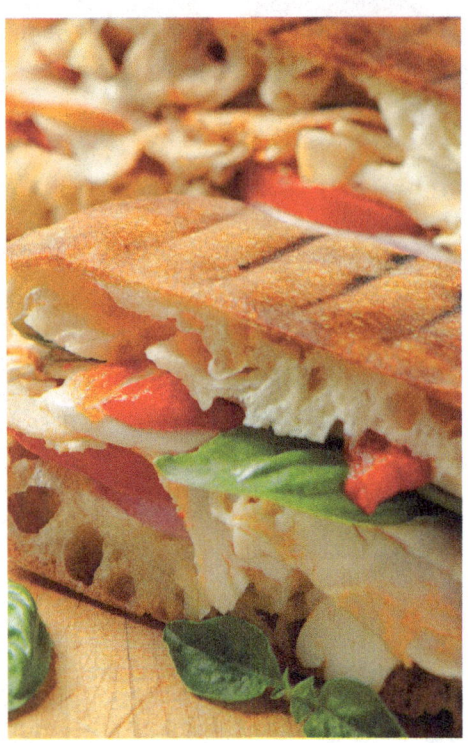

ITALIAN PANINI WITH PROVOLONE, PEPPERS, AND ARUGULA

Ingredients:
- 1/2 cup jarred roasted red peppers, drained
- 2 slices turkey (optional sub)
- 1/4 cup pitted kalamata olives
- 1 tablespoon olive oil
- 1 teaspoon balsamic vinegar
- Salt and black pepper to taste
- 4 slices whole wheat bread
- 4 slices provolone cheese
- 1 cup arugula leaves

Instructions:
1. Preheat oven to 350 degrees F.
2. In a medium bowl, mix together roasted red peppers, kalamata olives, olive oil, balsamic vinegar, salt and black pepper to taste. Set aside.
3. Place bread on a baking sheet and top with sliced cheese. Bake in preheated oven for 5-7 minutes, or until cheese is melted and bread is toasted.
4. Remove from oven and top with roasted pepper mixture and arugula leaves. Slice into 4 pieces and serve immediately.

Serving Size: 1 sandwich
Calories: 390

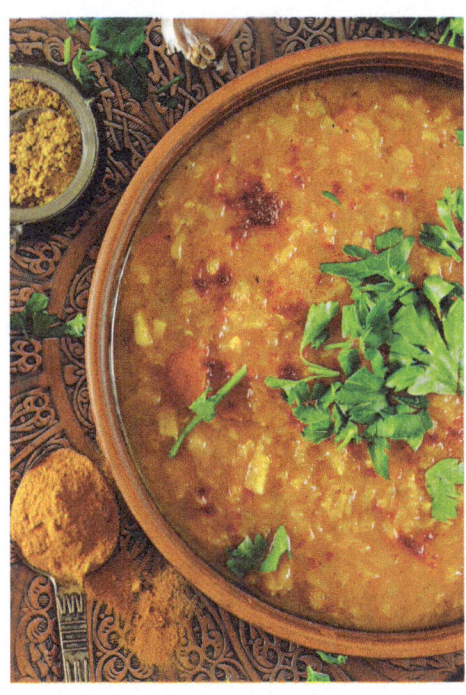

CURRIED LENTIL SOUP

Ingredients:

- 1 tablespoon olive oil
- 1 onion, diced
- 3 cloves garlic, minced
- 1 teaspoon grated ginger root
- 1 tablespoon curry powder
- 2 cups vegetable broth
- 1 cup dry lentils, rinsed and drained
- 1 can (15 ounces) diced tomatoes, undrained
- 1 can (15 ounces) chickpeas, rinsed and drained
- Salt and black pepper to taste

Instructions:

1. In a large pot or Dutch oven, heat olive oil over medium heat. Add onion, garlic, and ginger root and cook until onions are translucent.
2. Stir in curry powder and cook for 1 minute.
3. Add vegetable broth, lentils, diced tomatoes with their juice, and chickpeas. Season with salt and black pepper to taste. Bring to a boil.
4. Reduce heat to low and simmer for 30 minutes, or until lentils are cooked through. Serve immediately!

Serving Size: 1 bowl
Calories: 440

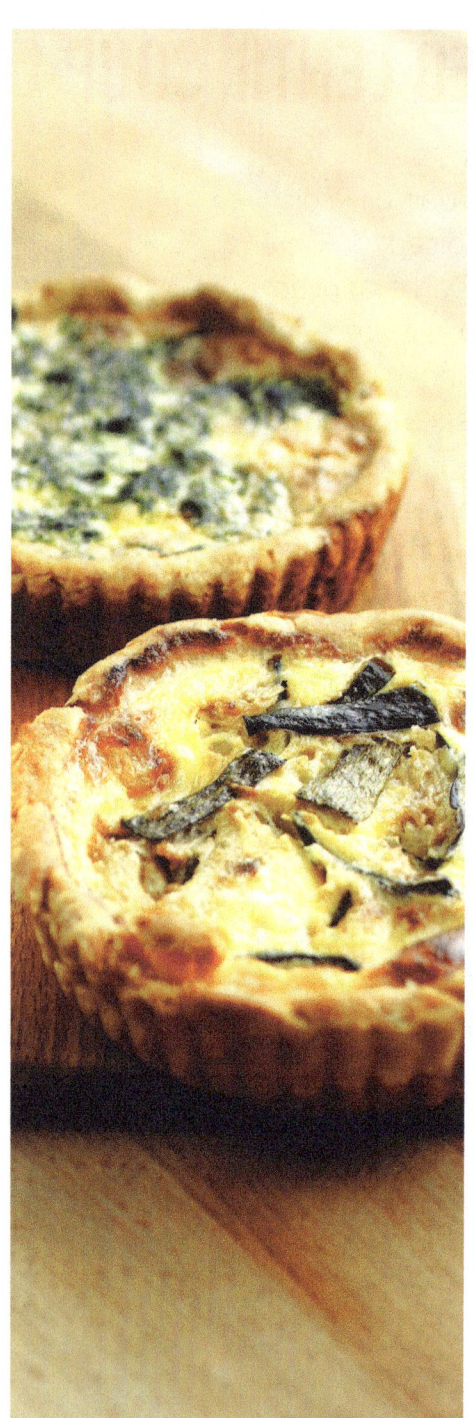

ARTICHOKE-FETA QUICHE

Ingredients:

- 1 unbaked 9-inch pie crust
- 1 tablespoon olive oil
- 1/2 onion, diced
- 3 cloves garlic, minced
- 1 can (14 ounces) artichoke hearts, drained and chopped
- 4 eggs
- 3/4 cup milk or non-dairy milk
- 1/2 teaspoon salt
- 1/4 teaspoon black pepper
- 1 cup shredded cheese or dairy-free cheese substitute
- 2 tablespoons crumbled feta cheese or dairy-free feta cheese substitute

Instructions:
1. Preheat oven to 375 degrees F.
2. In a large skillet, heat olive oil over medium heat. Add onion and garlic and cook until onions are translucent.
3. Stir in artichoke hearts and cook for 5 minutes.
4. In a large bowl, whisk together eggs, milk, salt, and black pepper. Stir in cooked artichoke mixture and shredded cheese. Pour into prepared pie crust. Sprinkle with crumbled feta cheese.
5. Bake in preheated oven for 30-35 minutes, or until quiche is firm in the center and the crust is golden brown. Let cool for 10 minutes before serving. Enjoy!

Serving Size: 1 slice
Calories: 380

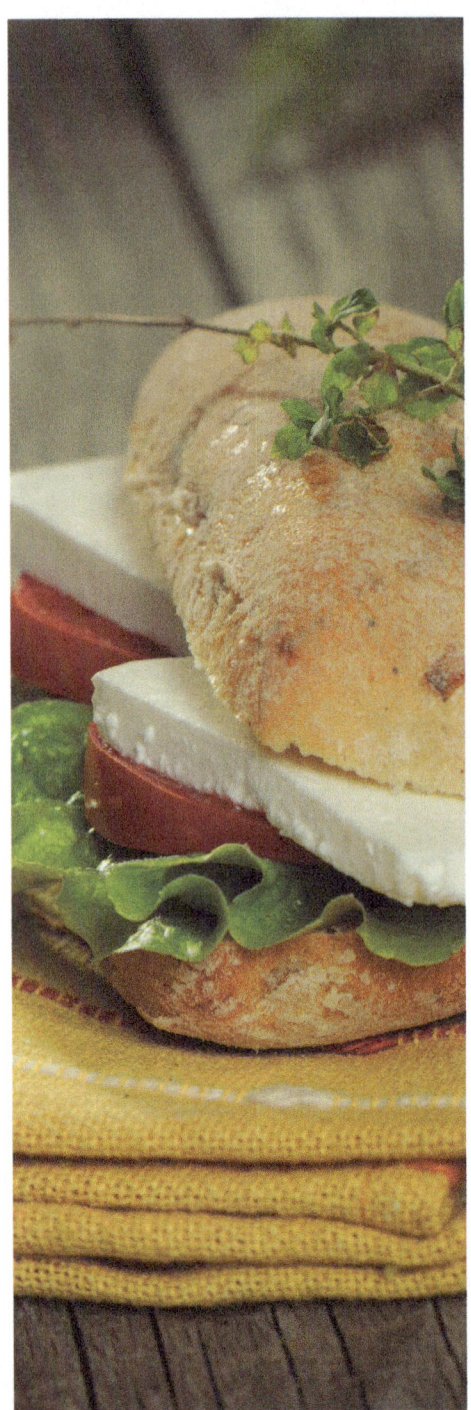

CAPRESE SANDWICH

Ingredients:
- 1/4 pound thinly sliced mozzarella cheese
- 1/4 pound thinly sliced fresh tomatoes
- 8 leaves fresh basil
- 1 tablespoon olive oil
- Salt and black pepper to taste
- 4 slices whole wheat bread

Instructions:
1. Preheat oven to 350 degrees F.
2. On a large baking sheet, alternate layering slices of mozzarella cheese, fresh tomatoes, and basil leaves. Drizzle with olive oil and season with salt and black pepper to taste.
3. Bake in preheated oven for 10-15 minutes, or until cheese is melted and bubbly and bread is toasted. Serve immediately!

Serving Size: 1 sandwich
Calories: 440

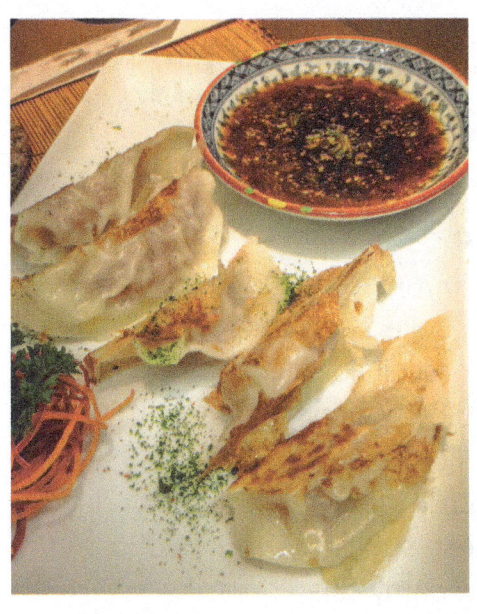

CHICKEN POT STICKERS

Ingredients:
- 1/2 pound ground chicken
- 1/4 cup shredded carrots
- 1/4 cup minced onion
- 2 cloves garlic, minced
- 1 teaspoon grated ginger root
- 1 tablespoon soy sauce or gluten-free tamari
- 1 teaspoon sesame oil
- 20 wonton wrappers or gluten-free wonton wrappers

Instructions:
1. In a large bowl, mix together ground chicken, carrots, onion, garlic, ginger root, soy sauce or tamari, and sesame oil.
2. To assemble pot stickers, place 1 tablespoon of the chicken mixture in the center of each wonton wrapper. Wet the edges of the wrapper with water and fold over to create a half-moon shape. Press the edges to seal.
3. In a large skillet or wok, heat 1 tablespoon of oil over medium-high heat. Add pot stickers and cook for 2-3 minutes per side, or until golden brown and crispy. Serve with your favorite dipping sauce!

Serving Size: 5 pot stickers
Calories: 210

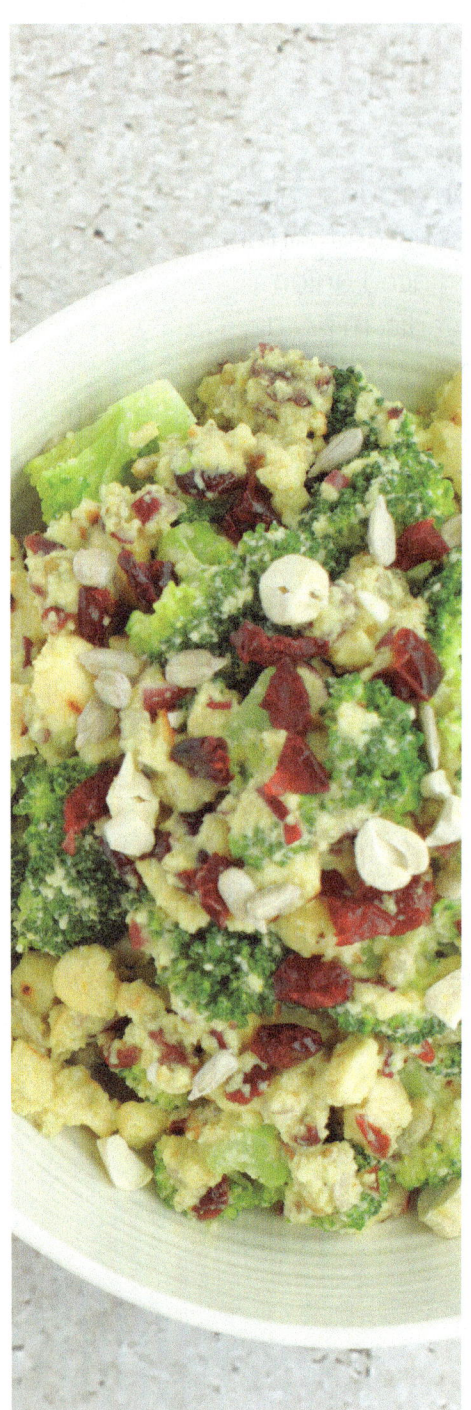

CHOPPED CHICKEN AND BROCCOLI SALAD

Ingredients:

- 1 pound boneless, skinless chicken breasts, cooked and chopped
- 3 cups broccoli florets, cooked
- 1/2 cup diced celery
- 1/2 cup diced red grapes
- 1/4 cup crumbled blue cheese or dairy-free cheese substitute
- 1/4 cup creamy salad dressing or Greek yogurt

Instructions:

1.. In a large bowl, mix together cooked chicken, broccoli, celery, grapes, blue cheese or cheese substitute, and salad dressing or mayonnaise.
2. Serve immediately or refrigerate until ready to eat. Enjoy!

Serving Size: 1 bowl
Calories: 490

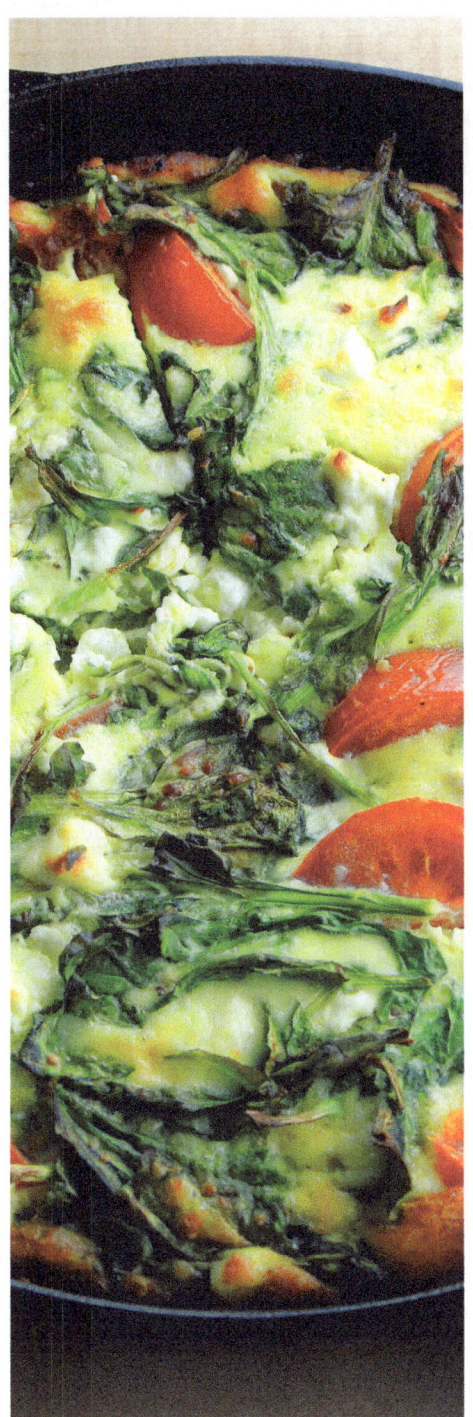

GREEN FRITTATA

Ingredients:
- 1 tablespoon olive oil
- 1/2 onion, diced
- 3 cloves garlic, minced
- 6 cups chopped spinach or kale
- 6 eggs
- 3/4 cup non-dairy milk
- 1/2 teaspoon salt
- 1/4 teaspoon black pepper

Instructions:
1. Preheat oven to 375 degrees F.
2. In a large skillet, heat olive oil over medium heat. Add onion and garlic and cook until onions are translucent.
3. Stir in chopped spinach or kale and cook until wilted.
4. In a large bowl, whisk together eggs, milk, salt, and black pepper. Stir in cooked vegetable mixture. Pour into prepared pie crust. Sprinkle with crumbled feta cheese.
5. Bake in preheated oven for 30-35 minutes, or until quiche is firm in the center and the crust is golden brown. Let cool for 10 minutes before serving. Enjoy!

Serving Size: 1 slice
Calories: 190

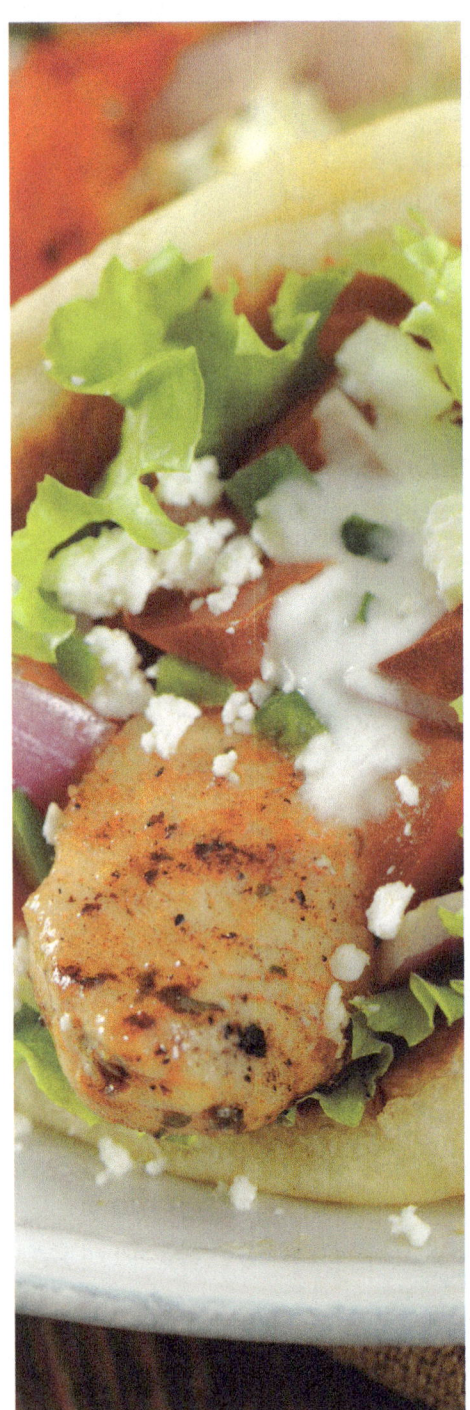

MEDITERRANEAN CHICKEN WRAP

Ingredients:
- 1 whole wheat tortilla
- 1/4 cup hummus
- 1/2 roasted chicken breast, shredded or chopped
- 1/4 cup diced cucumber
- 1/4 cup diced tomatoes
- 1 tablespoon crumbled feta cheese or dairy-free cheese substitute

Instructions:
1. Spread a layer of hummus on the tortilla.
2. Top with shredded chicken, cucumber, tomatoes, and feta cheese or cheese substitute. Roll up the tortilla and enjoy!

Serving Size: 1 wrap
Calories: 440

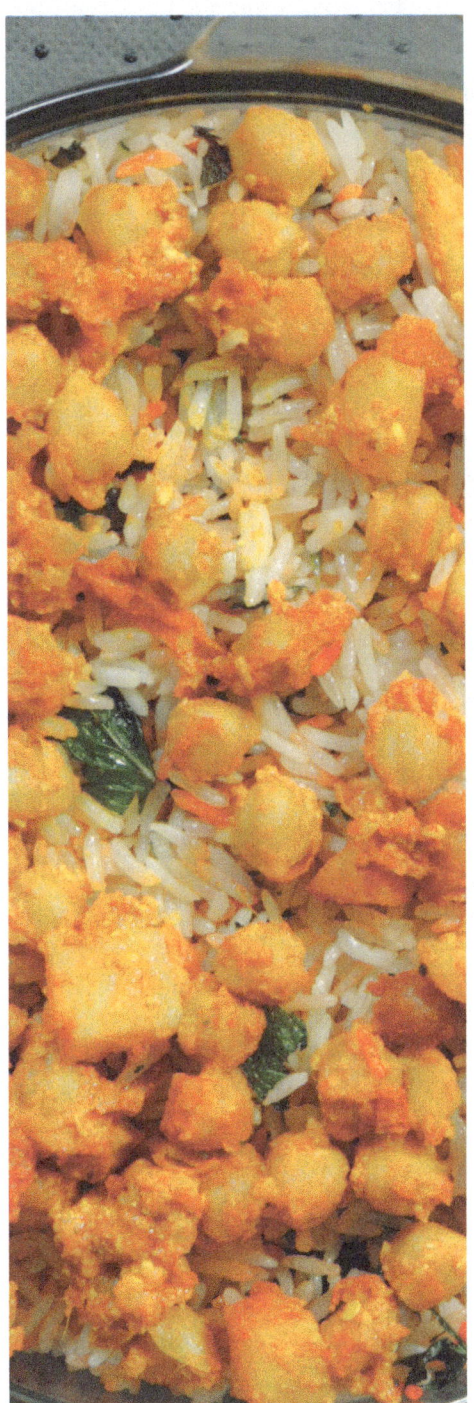

INSTANT POT PAKISTANI CHANA DAL

Ingredients:

- 1 cup chana dal or yellow split peas
- 4 cups water
- 1 teaspoon salt
- 1 tablespoon olive oil
- 1 onion, chopped
- 3 cloves garlic, minced
- 2 teaspoons cumin seeds
- 2 bay leaves
- 1 cinnamon stick
- 1 teaspoon turmeric powder
- 2 teaspoons ground coriander
- 1 (15-ounce) can diced tomatoes, undrained

Instructions:

1. In the Instant Pot, combine chana dal or yellow split peas, water, and salt. Stir well.
2. Close the lid and set the valve to sealing. Cook on high pressure for 30 minutes. When the cycle is complete, do a quick release of the pressure.
3. In a large skillet, heat olive oil over medium heat. Add onion and garlic and cook until onions are translucent.
4. Stir in cumin seeds, bay leaves, cinnamon stick, turmeric powder, and ground coriander. Cook for 1 minute longer.
5. Add the cooked dal or yellow split peas and diced tomatoes (undrained). Stir well and cook for 5 minutes longer, or until heated through. Serve immediately with rice or naan bread. Enjoy!

Serving Size: 1 bowl
Calories: 390

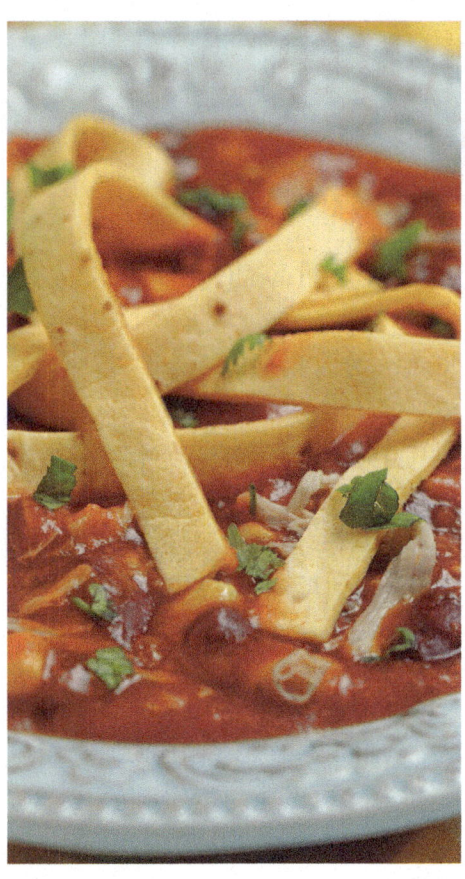

CHICKEN TORTILLA SOUP

Ingredients:
- 1 tablespoon olive oil
- 1 onion, diced
- 3 cloves garlic, minced
- 1 pound boneless, skinless chicken breasts, cooked and shredded
- 1 (14.5-ounce) can diced tomatoes, undrained
- 1 (4-ounce can diced green chilies, undrained)
- 2 cups chicken broth
- 1 teaspoon ground cumin
- 1 teaspoon chili powder
- 1/2 teaspoon salt
- 1/4 teaspoon black pepper

Instructions:
1. In a large pot or Dutch oven, heat olive oil over medium heat. Add onion and garlic and cook until onions are translucent.
2. Stir in cooked chicken, diced tomatoes with their juice, green chilies, chicken broth, cumin, chili powder, salt, and black pepper. Bring to a simmer and cook for 10 minutes.
3. Ladle soup into bowls and enjoy!

Serving Size: 1 bowl
Calories: 310

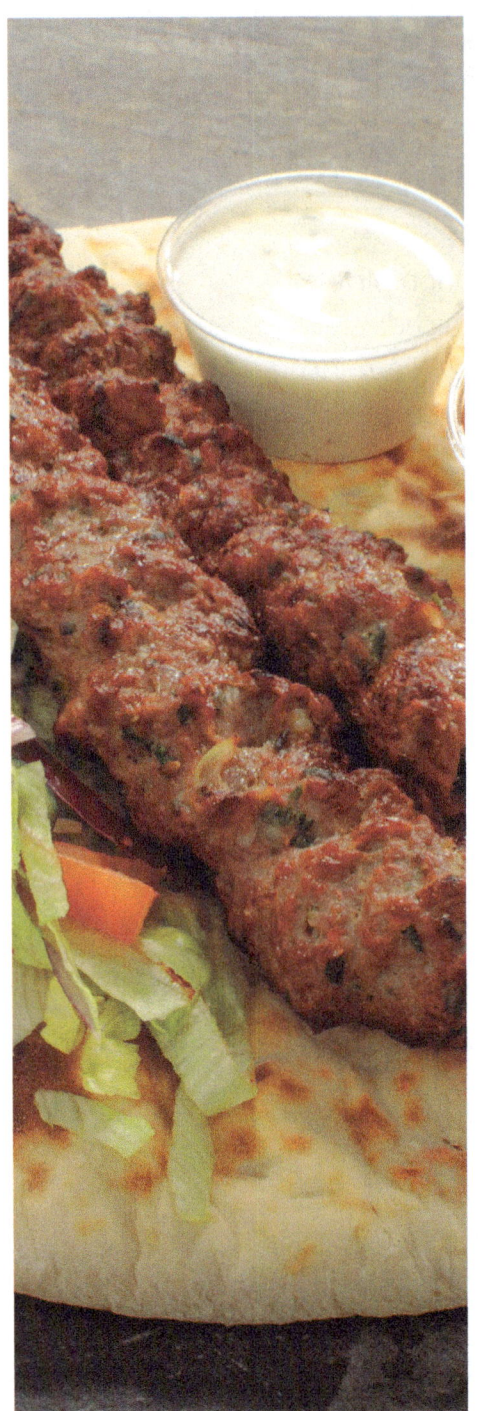

CHARGRILLED LAMB AND VEGGIE SANDWICH

Ingredients:
- 1/2 pound lamb, thinly sliced
- 1/2 teaspoon salt
- 1/4 teaspoon black pepper
- 1 tablespoon olive oil, divided
- 1 zucchini, thinly sliced lengthwise
- 1 red onion, thinly sliced
- 2 whole wheat tortillas
- 1/4 cup tzatziki sauce or plain yogurt

Instructions:
1. Preheat grill to medium-high heat.
2. Season lamb with salt and pepper. Grill for 3-4 minutes per side, or until cooked through. Remove from grill and chop into bite-sized pieces.
3. In a large skillet, heat 1 tablespoon olive oil over medium heat. Add zucchini and onion slices and cook until tender, stirring occasionally.
4. To assemble the sandwiches, spread each tortilla with tzatziki sauce or yogurt. Top with grilled lamb and veggies. Roll up and enjoy!

Serving Size: 1 sandwich
Calories: 420

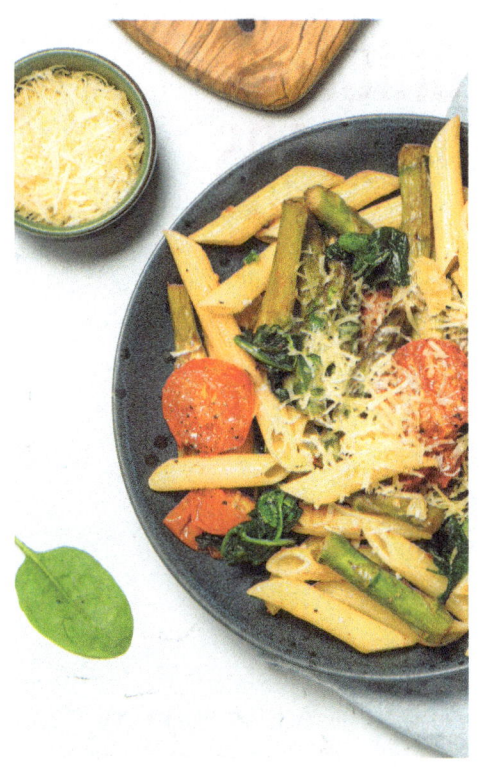

VEGAN SPINACH AND SUN-DRIED TOMATO PASTA

Ingredients:

- 8 ounces whole wheat pasta
- 1 tablespoon olive oil
- 3 cloves garlic, minced
- 1 (10-ounce) package frozen chopped spinach, thawed and squeezed of excess water
- 1/2 cup sun-dried tomatoes, packed in oil and drained
- 1/4 teaspoon salt
- 1/4 teaspoon black pepper

Instructions:

1. Cook pasta according to package instructions.
2. In a large skillet, heat olive oil over medium heat. Add garlic and cook until fragrant.
3. Stir in spinach, sun-dried tomatoes, salt, and black pepper. Cook for 5 minutes, or until heated through.
4. Drain pasta and add it to the skillet with the spinach and sun-dried tomatoes. Toss to combine. Serve immediately. Enjoy!

Serving Size: 1 bowl
Calories: 380

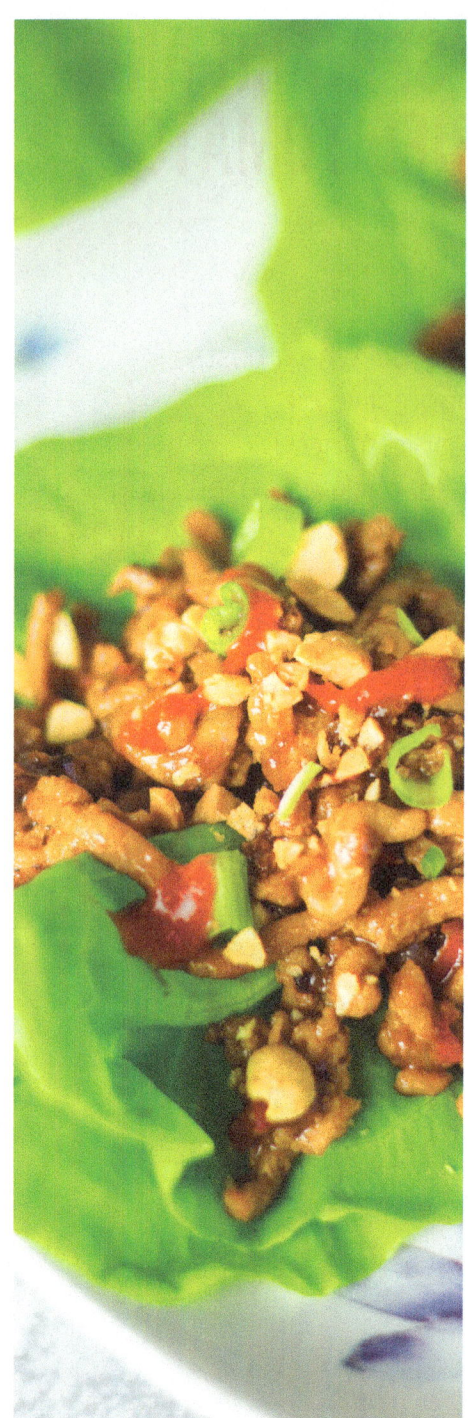

ASIAN CHICKEN LETTUCE WRAPS

Ingredients:

- 1 tablespoon sesame oil
- 1 pound ground chicken
- 1/2 cup chopped onion
- 3 cloves garlic, minced
- 1/4 cup hoisin sauce
- 1 tablespoon rice vinegar
- 1 teaspoon ground ginger

Instructions:

1. In a large skillet, heat sesame oil over medium-high heat. Add ground chicken, onion, and garlic. Cook until chicken is browned and cooked through.
2. Stir in hoisin sauce, rice vinegar, and ginger. Cook for 1 minute longer, or until heated through.
3. Serve chicken mixture on lettuce leaves and enjoy!

Serving Size: 1 wrap
Calories: 260

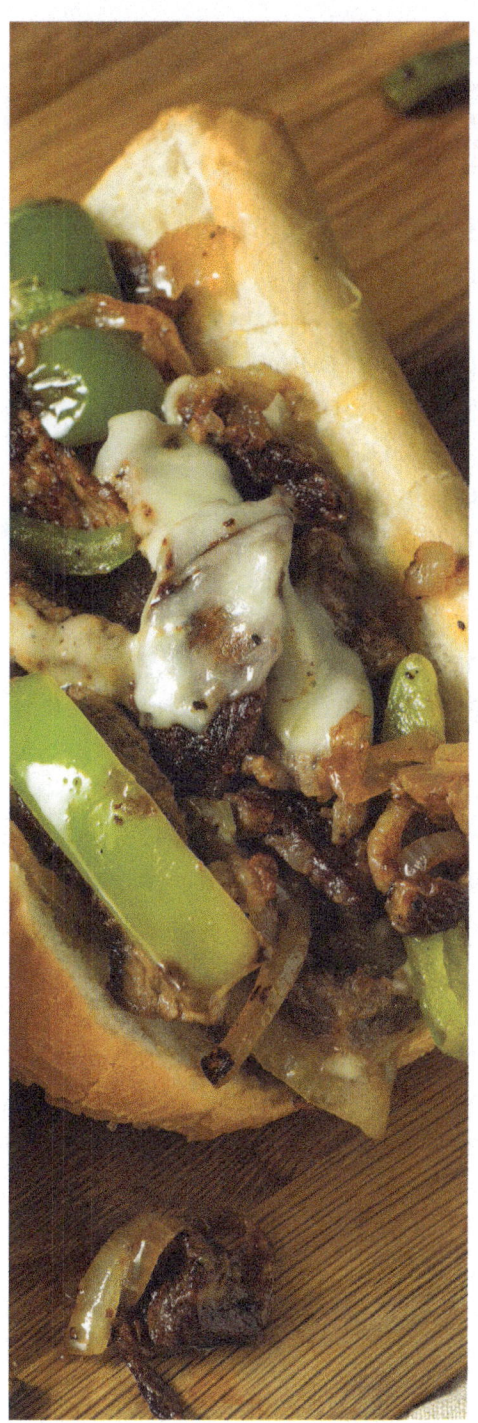

PORTOBELLO CHEESESTEAK

Ingredients:
- 1 tablespoon olive oil
- 2 large portobello mushroom caps, thinly sliced
- 1/2 onion, thinly sliced
- 1 green pepper, thinly sliced
- 1/4 teaspoon salt
- 1/4 teaspoon black pepper

Instructions:
1. In a large skillet, heat olive oil over medium-high heat. Add mushrooms, onion, and green pepper. Cook until vegetables are tender, stirring occasionally.
2. Season with salt and black pepper. Serve on whole wheat rolls and enjoy!

Serving Size: 1 sandwich
Calories: 320

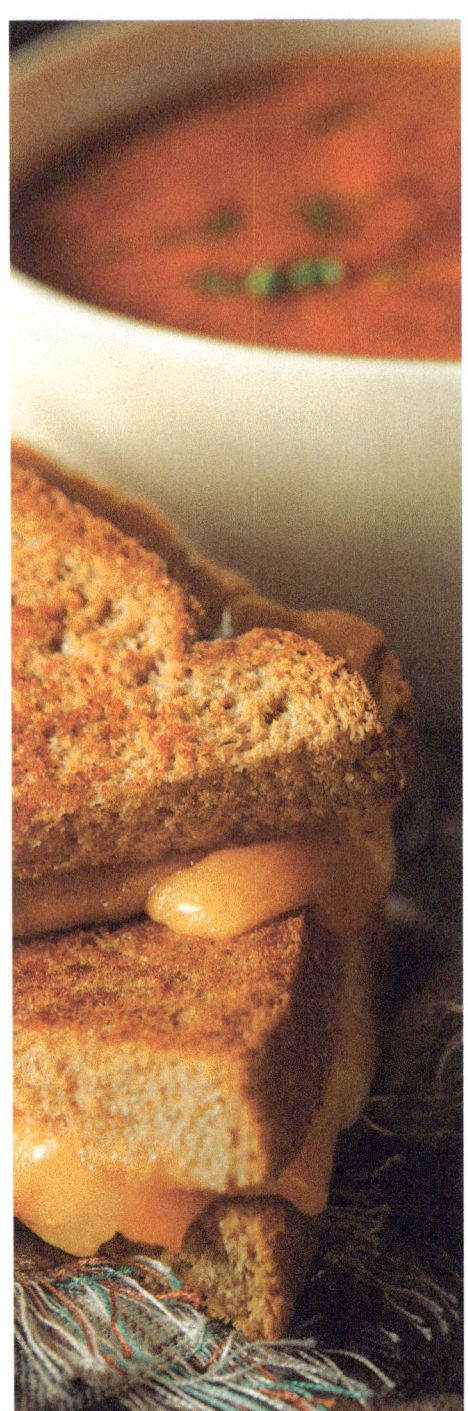

GRILLED CHEESE AND TOMATO SOUP

Ingredients:

- 1 tablespoon olive oil
- 2 cloves garlic, minced
- 2 tablespoons all-purpose flour
- 4 cups vegetable broth
- 1 (14.5-ounce) can diced tomatoes, undrained
- 1/4 teaspoon salt
- 1/4 teaspoon black pepper

Instructions:

1. In a large pot or Dutch oven, heat olive oil over medium heat. Add garlic and cook until fragrant.
2. Stir in flour and cook for 1 minute. Slowly whisk in vegetable broth until no lumps remain.
3. Add diced tomatoes and bring to a simmer. Cook for 10 minutes, or until heated through. Season with salt and black pepper.
4. Serve soup with grilled cheese sandwiches and enjoy!

Serving Size: 1 bowl
Calories: 440

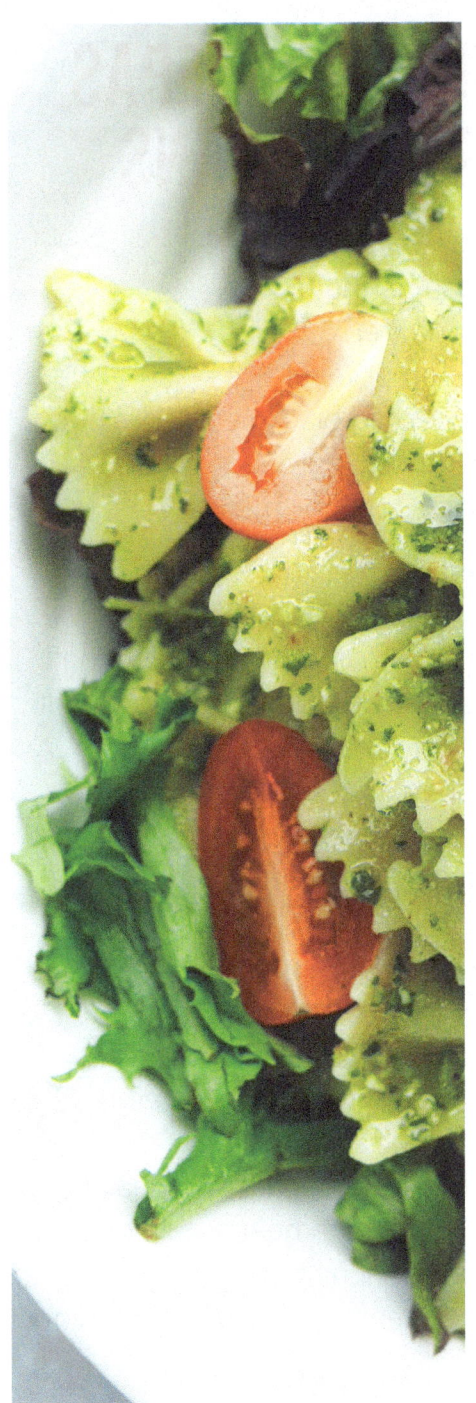

PASTA SALAD WITH LENTILS, PESTO, AND BEANS

Ingredients:
- 8 ounces whole wheat pasta
- 1/2 cup cooked lentils
- 1/4 cup pesto
- 1 (15-ounce) can kidney beans, drained and rinsed
- 1/2 cup diced tomatoes

Instructions:
1. Cook pasta according to package instructions.
2. In a large bowl, combine cooked pasta, lentils, pesto, kidney beans, and diced tomatoes. Toss to combine. Serve immediately or refrigerate for later. Enjoy!

Serving Size: 1 salad
Calories: 290

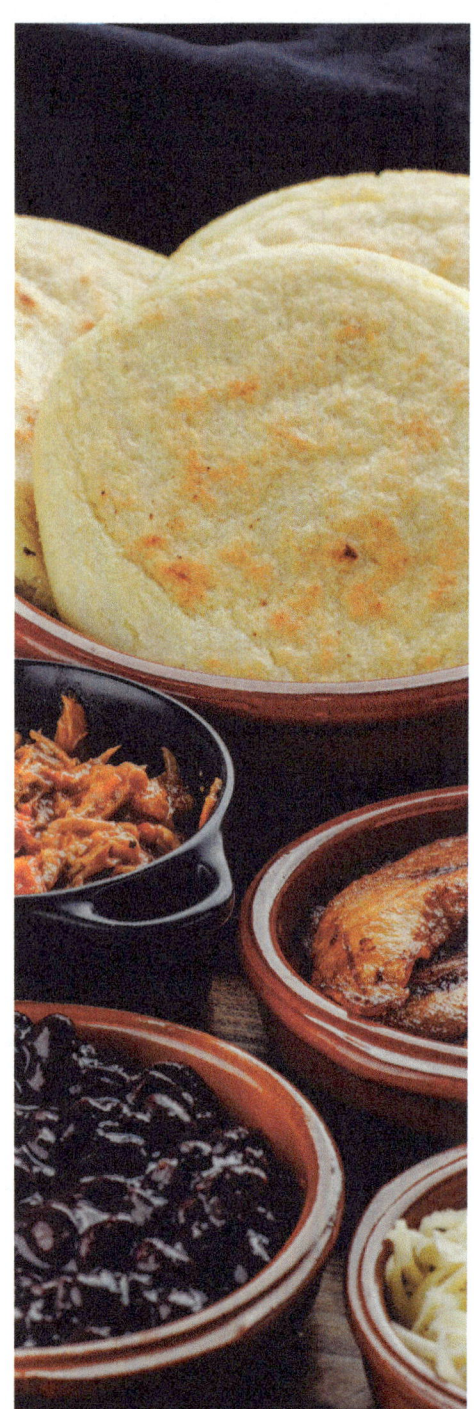

VENEZUELAN AREPAS WITH BLACK BEANS

Ingredients:

- 1 cup masa harina
- 1 1/2 cups water
- 1 tablespoon olive oil
- 1 (15-ounce) can black beans, drained and rinsed
- 1/4 cup diced onion

Instructions:

1. Preheat oven to 375 degrees F.
2. In a large bowl, combine masa harina and water. Mix until well combined. Let dough sit for 5 minutes.
3. Divide dough into 8 equal pieces and shape into balls. Flatten each ball into a disc shape.
4. In a large skillet, heat olive oil over medium heat. Add arepas and cook for 2 minutes per side, or until golden brown.
5. Transfer arepas to a baking sheet and bake for 10 minutes.
6. In the same skillet, heat black beans and onion over medium heat. Cook for 5 minutes, or until heated through.
7. Serve black beans on arepas and enjoy!

Serving Size: 2 arepas
Calories: 380

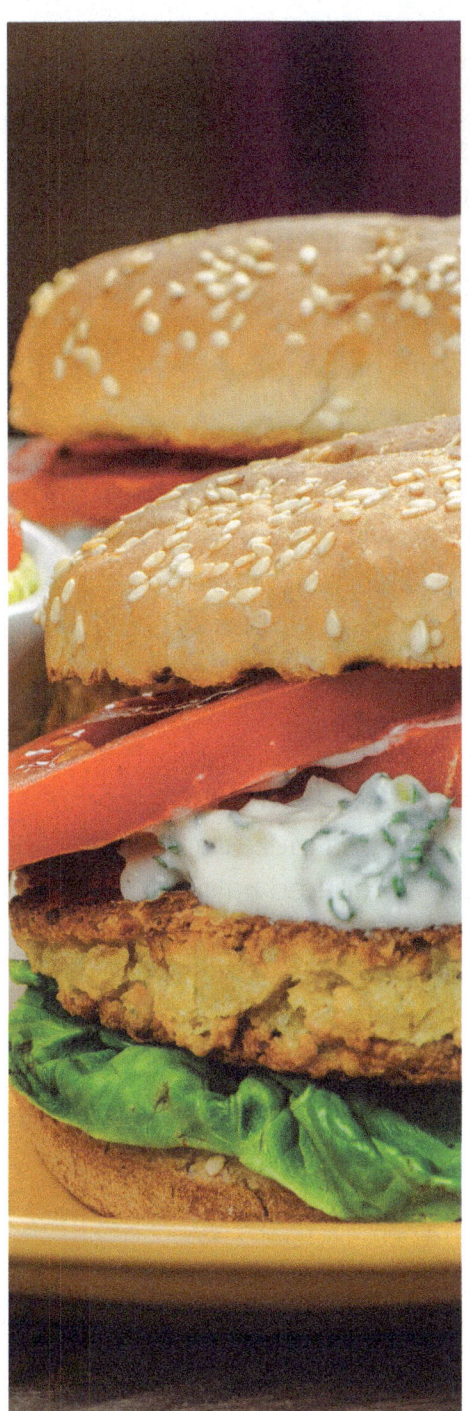

GARLIC CHILI CHICKPEA PATTIES

Ingredients:

- 1 (15-ounce) can chickpeas, drained and rinsed
- 3 cloves garlic, minced
- 1 teaspoon ground chili powder
- 1/4 teaspoon salt
- /4 teaspoon black pepper
- 2 tablespoons chopped fresh cilantro leaves

Instructions:

1. Preheat oven to 375 degrees F. Line a baking sheet with parchment paper.
2. In a large bowl, mash chickpeas until thick and pasty. Stir in garlic, chili powder, salt, black pepper, and cilantro. Mix until well combined.
3. Divide mixture into 8 equal patties and place on the prepared baking sheet. Bake for 20 minutes, or until golden brown. Serve immediately and enjoy!

Serving Size: 2 patties
Calories: 190

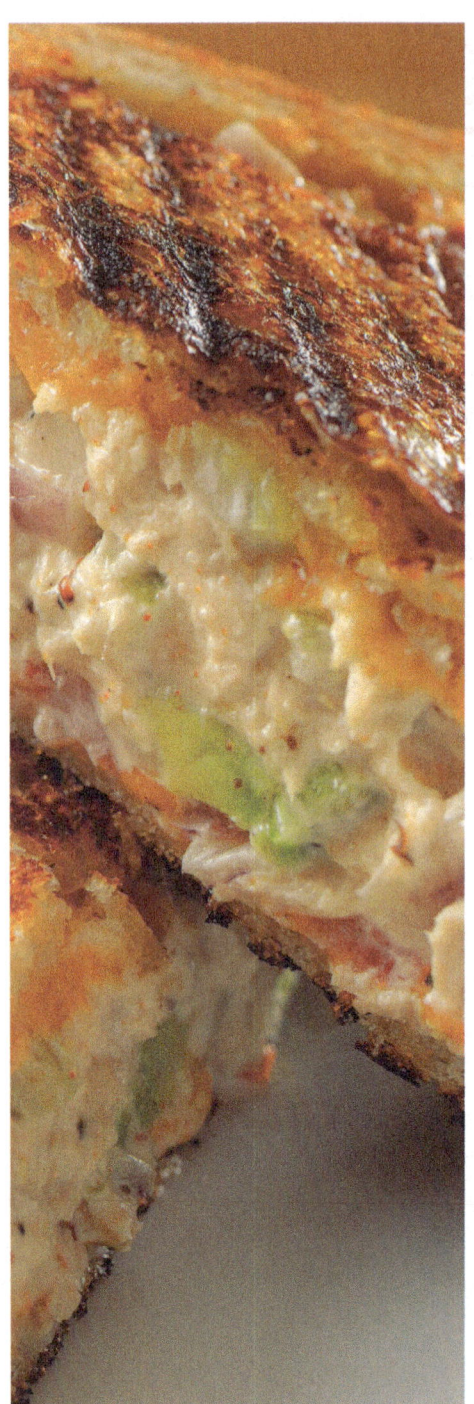

ITALIAN TUNA MELT

Ingredients:
- 2 tablespoons olive oil
- 4 cloves garlic, minced
- 1 (6-ounce) can tuna, drained
- 1/4 teaspoon salt
- 1/4 teaspoon black pepper

Instructions:
1. Preheat oven to 400 degrees F. Line a baking sheet with parchment paper.
2. In a small skillet, heat olive oil over medium heat. Add garlic and cook until fragrant. Stir in tuna and season with salt and black pepper. Cook for 2 minutes, or until heated through.
3. Place tuna on whole wheat bread and top with shredded mozzarella cheese. Place on the prepared baking sheet and bake for 10 minutes, or until cheese is melted and bubbly. Serve immediately. Enjoy!

Serving Size: 1 sandwich
Calories: 420

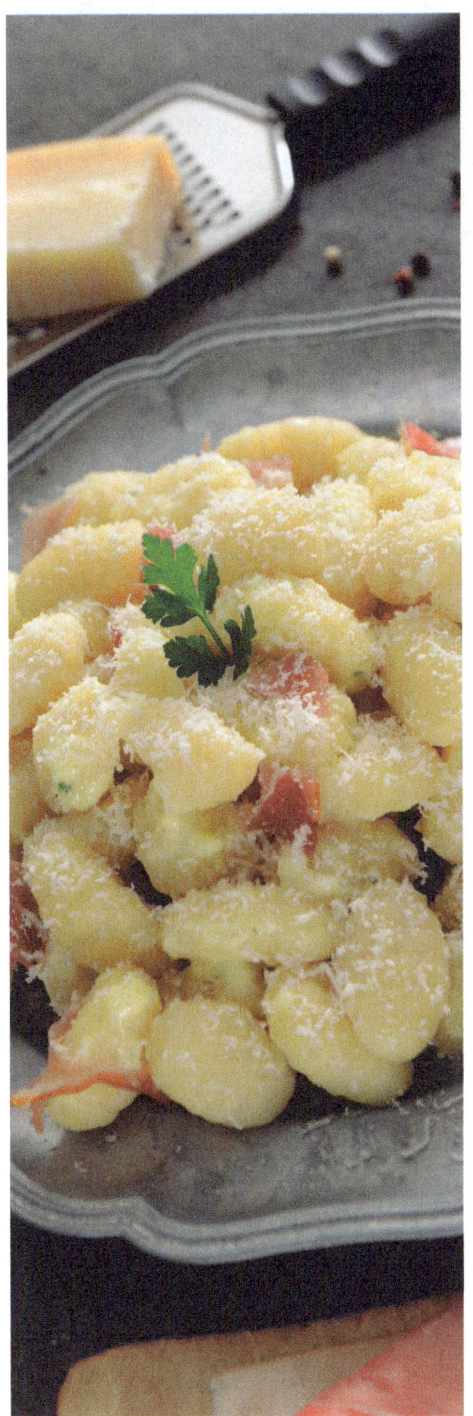

GNOCCHI WITH PEAS AND PROSCIUTTO

Ingredients:

- 1 (16-ounce) package shelf-stable gnocchi
- 1/4 cup diced onion
- 3 cloves garlic, minced
- 1/2 cup frozen peas
- 1/4 cup chopped prosciutto

Instructions:

1. In a large pot or Dutch oven, bring water to a boil. Add gnocchi and cook for 2 minutes, or until they float to the surface. Drain and set aside.
2. In the same pot, heat olive oil over medium heat. Add onion and garlic and cook until fragrant. Stir in frozen peas and cook for 2 minutes, or until heated through.
3. Add cooked gnocchi and prosciutto to the pot. Toss to combine and cook for 2 minutes, or until heated through. Serve immediately and enjoy!

Serving Size: 1 1/2 cups
Calories: 490

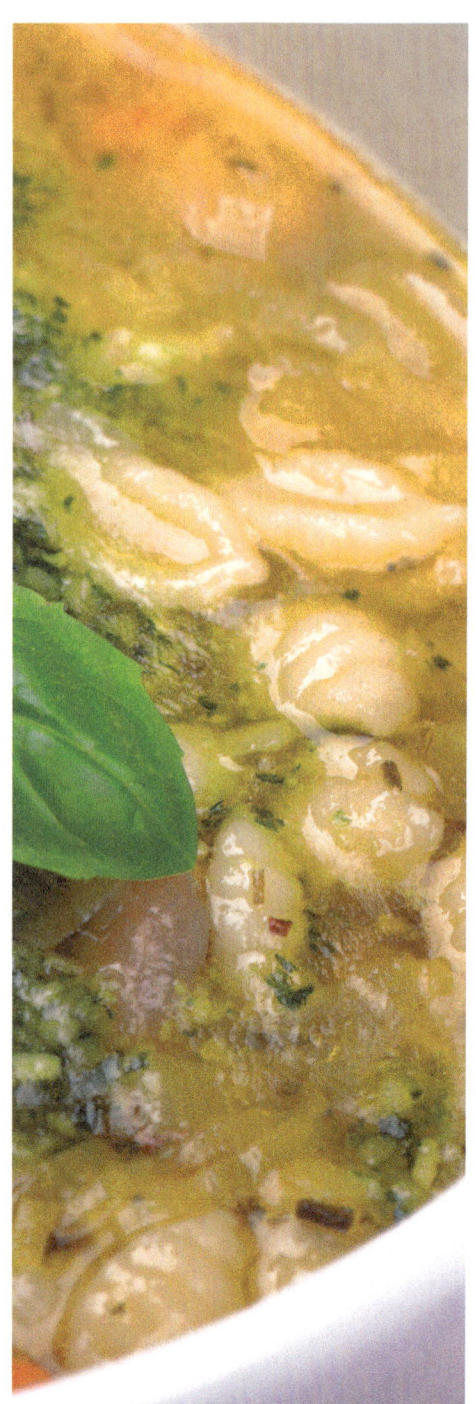

MINESTRONE WITH PESTO

Ingredients:
- 1 tablespoon olive oil
- 4 cloves garlic, minced
- 1/2 cup diced onion
- 3 cups vegetable broth
- 1 (15-ounce) can diced tomatoes, undrained
- 1 (15-ounce) can kidney beans, drained and rinsed
- 1 cup chopped fresh spinach leaves

Instructions:
1. In a large pot or Dutch oven, heat olive oil over medium heat. Add garlic and onion and cook until fragrant.
2. Stir in vegetable broth, diced tomatoes with their juice, kidney beans, and chopped spinach leaves. Bring to a boil.
3. Reduce heat to low and let soup simmer for 10 minutes. Serve immediately with a dollop of pesto and enjoy!

Serving Size: 1 1/2 cups
Calories: 310

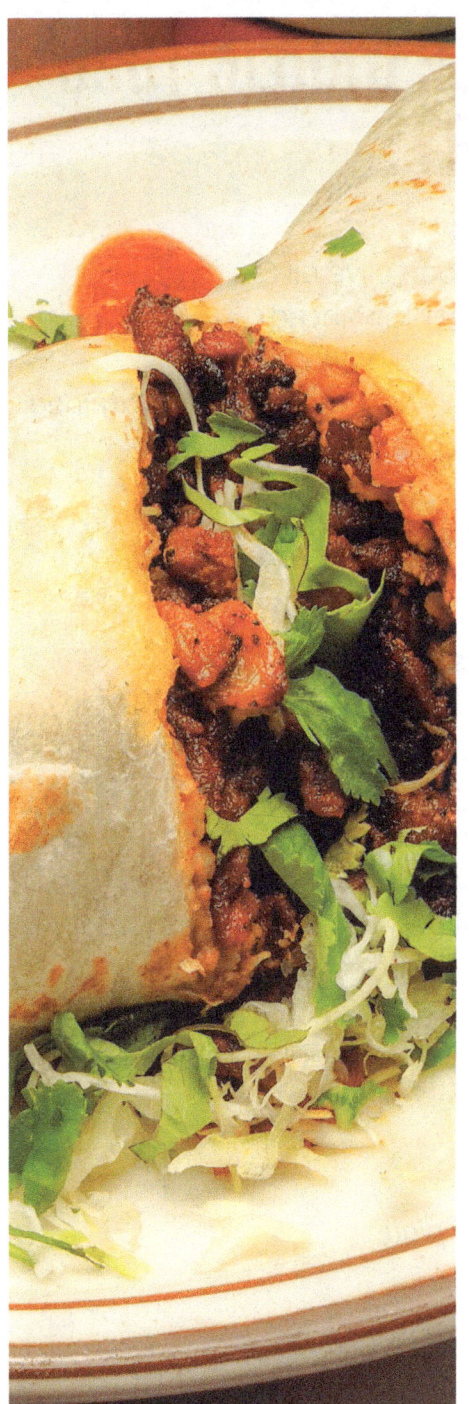

CARNE ASADA BURRITOS

Ingredients:

- 1 pound flank steak
- 1/4 teaspoon salt
- 1/4 teaspoon black pepper
- 1 tablespoon olive oil
- 1/2 cup diced onion
- 2 cloves garlic, minced
- 1 (14.5-ounce) can diced tomatoes, undrained

Instructions:

1. Season both sides of the steak with salt and black pepper. Heat a grill or grill pan over medium-high heat and cook the steak for 5 minutes per side, or until it reaches the desired level of doneness. Remove from heat and let rest for 5 minutes before slicing into thin strips.
2. In a large skillet, heat olive oil over medium heat. Add onion and garlic and cook until fragrant. Stir in diced tomatoes with their juice and the steak strips. Cook for 5 minutes, or until heated through.
3. Serve the steak mixture on whole wheat tortillas and enjoy!

Serving Size: 1 burrito
Calories: 490

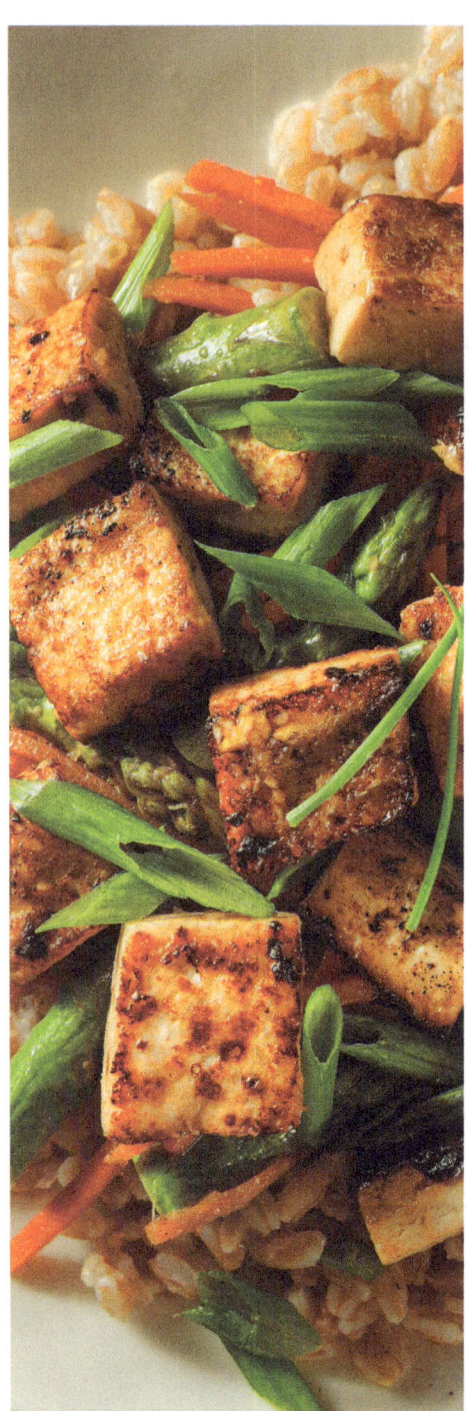

CHINESE GARLIC TOFU STIR FRY

Ingredients:
- 1 tablespoon olive oil
- 4 cloves garlic, minced
- 1/2 cup diced onion
- 1 (14-ounce) package firm tofu, drained and cubed
- 3/4 cup vegetable broth
- 1/4 cup low sodium soy sauce
- 1 tablespoon honey

Instructions:
1. In a large skillet or wok, heat olive oil over medium-high heat. Add garlic and onion and cook until fragrant.
2. Stir in tofu and cook for 5 minutes, or until browned.
3. In a small bowl, whisk together vegetable broth, soy sauce, and honey. Pour over the tofu mixture and cook for 3 minutes, or until heated through. Serve immediately with rice and enjoy!

Serving Size: 1 plate
Calories: 420

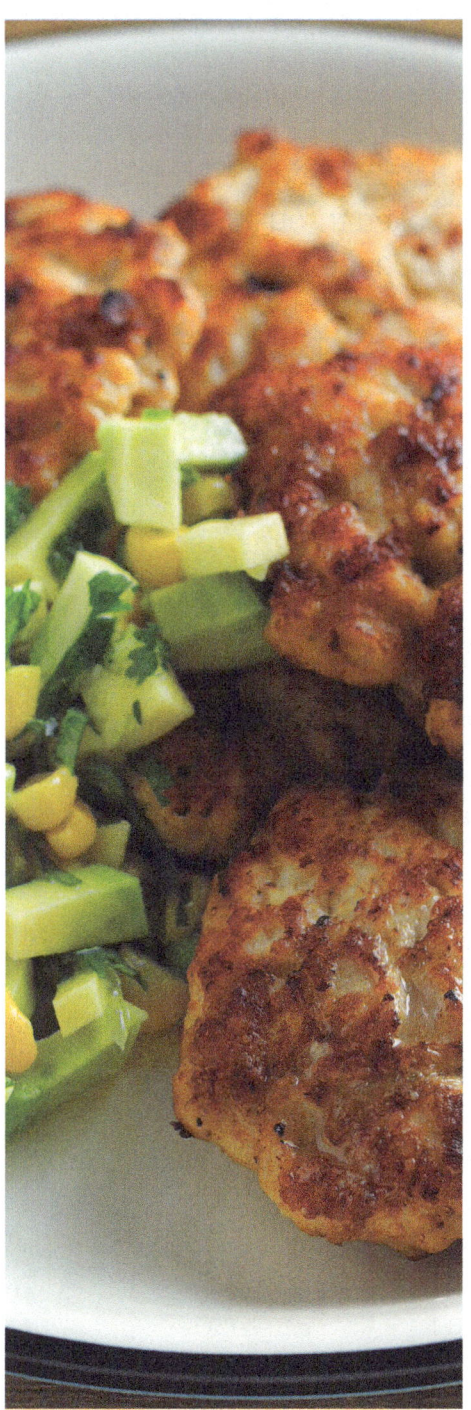

HEALTHY CRAB CAKES WITH MANGO-AVOCADO SALSA

Ingredients:
- 1/4 cup diced onion
- 2 cloves garlic, minced
- 1 pound fresh lump crabmeat
- 1/4 cup finely chopped fresh cilantro leaves
- 1 large egg, beaten
- 1 tablespoon low sodium soy sauce
- 1 tablespoon Dijon mustard

For the mango-avocado salsa:
- 1 ripe mango, peeled, seeded, and diced
- 1 ripe avocado, peeled, seeded, and diced
- 1 small jalapeno pepper, seeded and minced
- 2 tablespoons diced red onion
- 1 tablespoon fresh lime juice

Instructions:

1. In a large bowl, combine onion, garlic, crabmeat, cilantro, egg, soy sauce, and Dijon mustard. Mix well and shape into 8 patties.
2. Heat a grill or grill pan over medium-high heat and cook the crab cakes for 4 minutes per side, or until golden brown and cooked through.
3. In a medium bowl, combine mango, avocado, jalapeno pepper, red onion, and lime juice. Toss to combine.
4. Serve the crab cakes with the mango-avocado salsa and enjoy!

Serving Size: 2 crab cakes + 1/2 cup salsa
Calories: 400

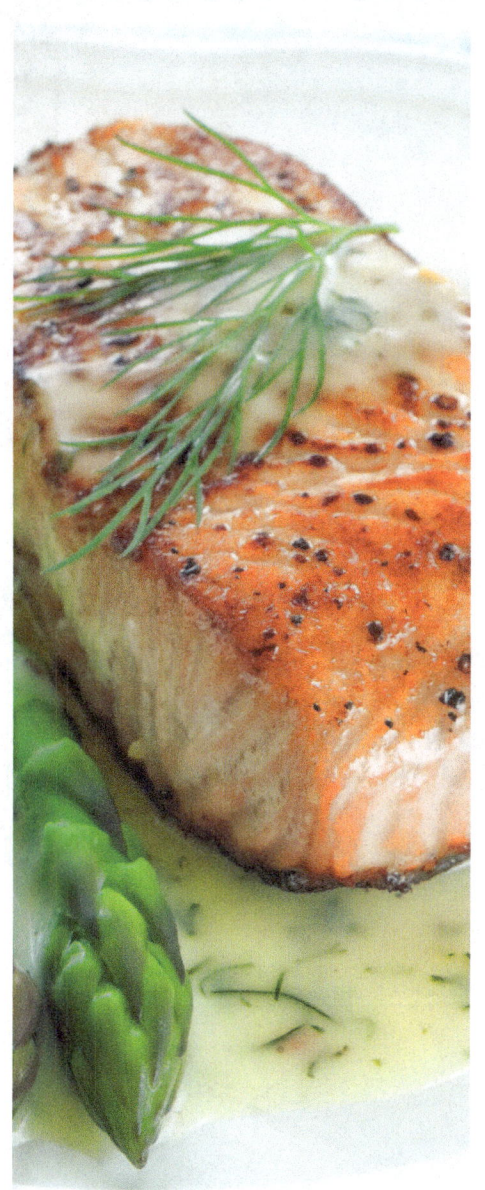

DILLED SALMON WITH ROASTED ASPARAGUS

Ingredients:
- 1 pound fresh salmon filets
- 1/4 teaspoon salt
- 1/4 teaspoon black pepper
- 1 tablespoon olive oil
- 1 bunch asparagus, trimmed

Instructions:
1. Preheat oven to 400 degrees F (200 degrees C).
2. Sprinkle both sides of the salmon filets with salt and black pepper. Heat a large skillet over medium-high heat and add olive oil. Add the salmon filets and cook for 3 minutes per side, or until golden brown. Remove from heat and set aside.
3. In the same skillet, add the asparagus. Cook for 5 minutes, or until tender.
4. Place the salmon and asparagus on a baking sheet and bake for 10 minutes, or until the salmon is cooked through. Serve immediately and enjoy!

Serving Size: 1 filet + 1/2 cup asparagus
Calories: 400

CHAPTER FIVE:

Dinners

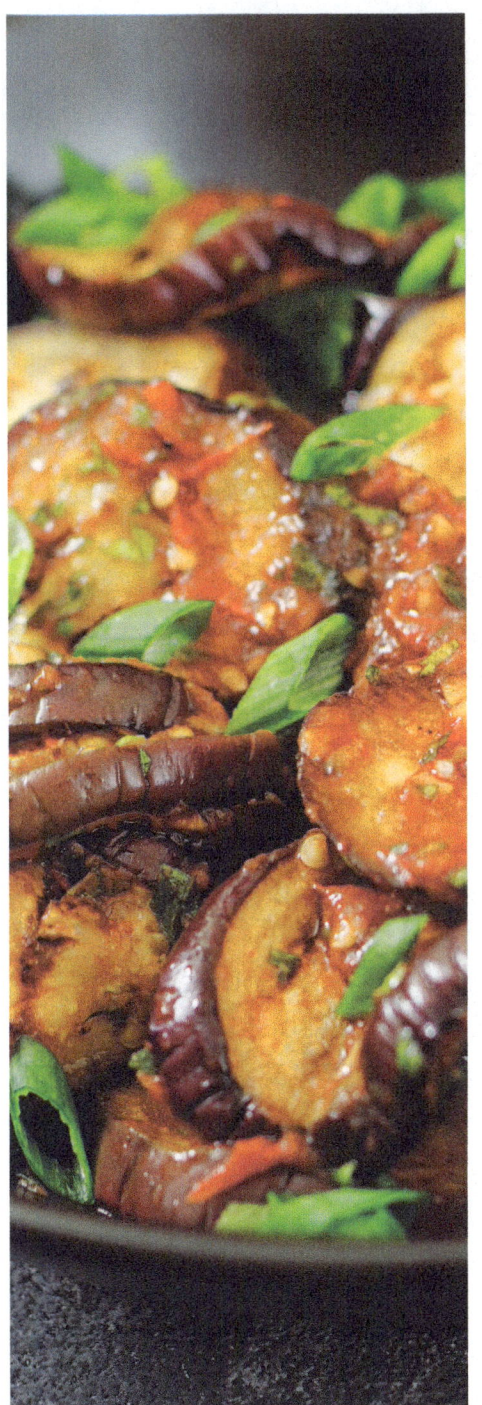

MISO-ROASTED EGGPLANT STEAKS WITH SWEET POTATOES

Ingredients:
- 2 large eggplants, sliced into 1-inch thick steaks
- 1/4 cup white miso paste
- 3 tablespoons tamari or soy sauce
- 3 tablespoons rice vinegar
- 3 tablespoons maple syrup
- 1 tablespoon sesame oil
- 3 cloves garlic, minced
- 1 teaspoon ground ginger

Instructions:
1. Preheat oven to 375 degrees F.
2. In a small bowl, whisk together miso paste, tamari or soy sauce, rice vinegar, maple syrup, sesame oil, garlic, and ginger.
3. Place eggplant steaks on a greased baking sheet and spread miso mixture over top. Bake for 25-30 minutes, or until eggplant is tender and miso mixture is nicely browned and bubbly. Serve immediately!

Serving Size: 1 eggplant steaks
Calories: 400

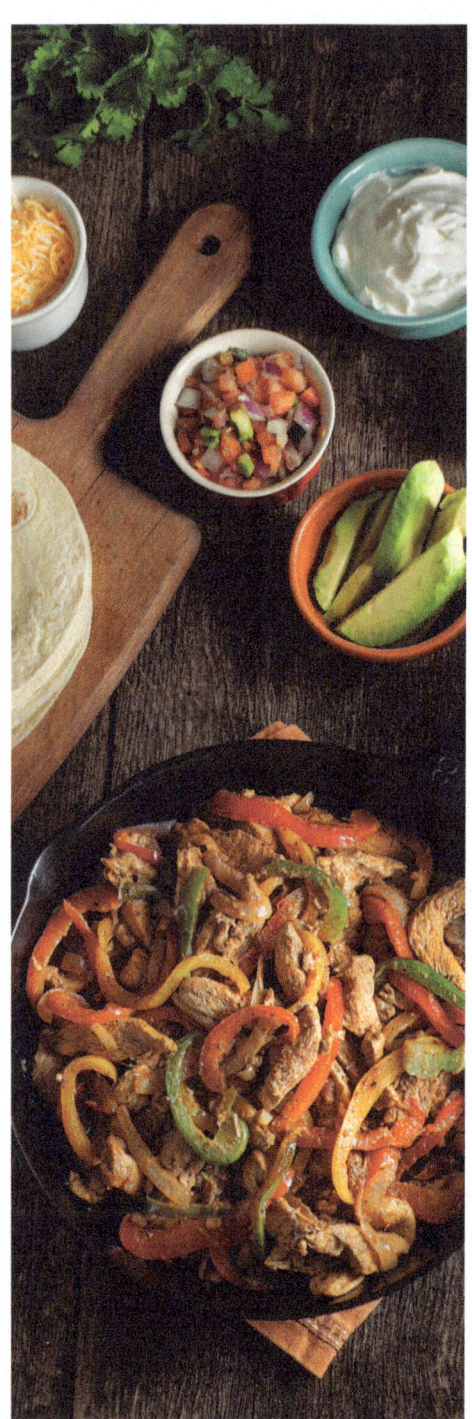

CHIPOTLE CHICKEN FAJITAS

Ingredients:

- 1 pound boneless, skinless chicken breasts, thinly sliced
- 1 red bell pepper, thinly sliced
- 1 yellow bell pepper, thinly sliced
- 1 orange bell pepper, thinly sliced
- 1/2 onion, thinly sliced
- 3 cloves garlic, minced
- 1 tablespoon chili powder
- 1 teaspoon ground cumin
- 1 teaspoon smoked paprika
- Salt and black pepper to taste

For the sauce:

- 1/2 cup plain non-dairy yogurt
- 1/4 cup chopped cilantro
- Juice of 1 lime
- 1 chipotle pepper in adobo sauce, plus 1 tablespoon of the sauce

Instructions:

1. In a large bowl, mix together chicken, bell peppers, onion, garlic, chili powder, cumin, smoked paprika, salt and black pepper.
2. In a small bowl, whisk together yogurt, cilantro, lime juice, chipotle pepper, and adobo sauce. Set aside.
3. Heat a large skillet over medium heat and spray with cooking spray. Add chicken mixture and cook for 5-7 minutes per side, or until chicken is cooked through and veggies are slightly charred.
4. Serve immediately with chipotle sauce!

Serving Size: 1 fajitas
Calories: 400

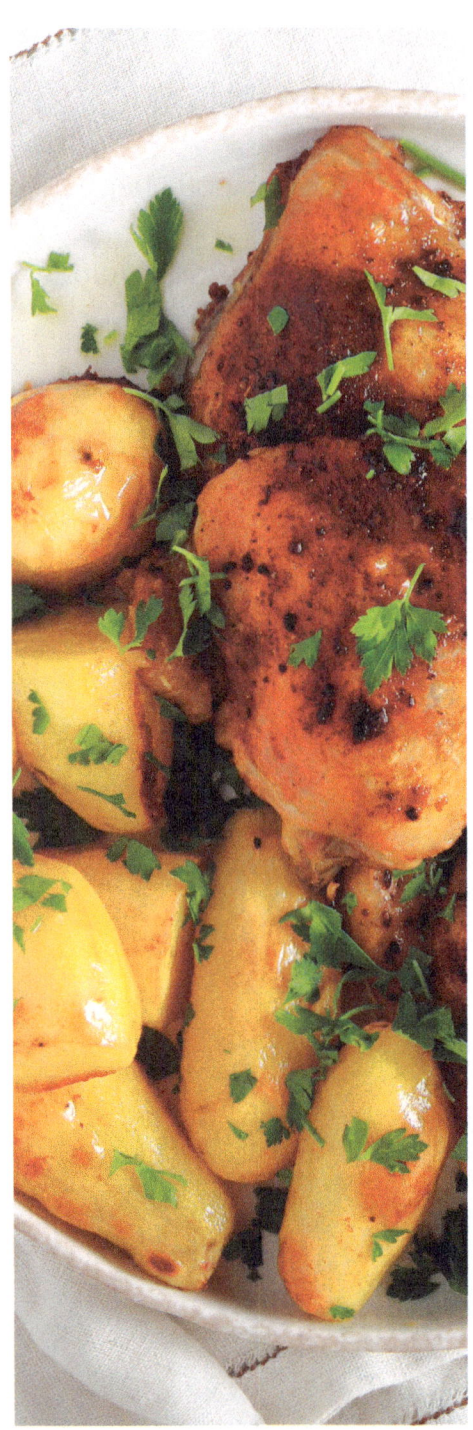

ROASTED CHICKEN AND POTATO WITH KALE SALAD

Ingredients:
- 1 pound boneless, skinless chicken breasts
- 1 pound Yukon gold potatoes, cut into 1-inch chunks
- 1/4 cup olive oil, divided
- Salt and black pepper to taste
- 3 cloves garlic, minced
- 1/4 teaspoon dried thyme
- 1/4 teaspoon dried oregano
- 1/4 teaspoon dried basil

For the salad:
- 3 cups chopped kale
- 1/4 cup diced red onion
- 1/4 cup diced avocado
- 2 tablespoons lemon juice

Instructions:
1. Preheat oven to 375 degrees F.
2. In a large bowl, mix together chicken, potatoes, 2 tablespoons of olive oil, salt and black pepper, garlic, thyme, oregano, and basil.
3. Spread mixture onto a greased baking sheet and roast for 25-30 minutes, or until chicken is cooked through and potatoes are tender and slightly browned.
4. In a large bowl, mix together kale, onion, avocado, lemon juice, and remaining 2 tablespoons of olive oil. Season with salt and black pepper to taste.
5. Serve roasted chicken and potatoes with kale salad on the side!

Serving Size: 1 plate
Calories: 520

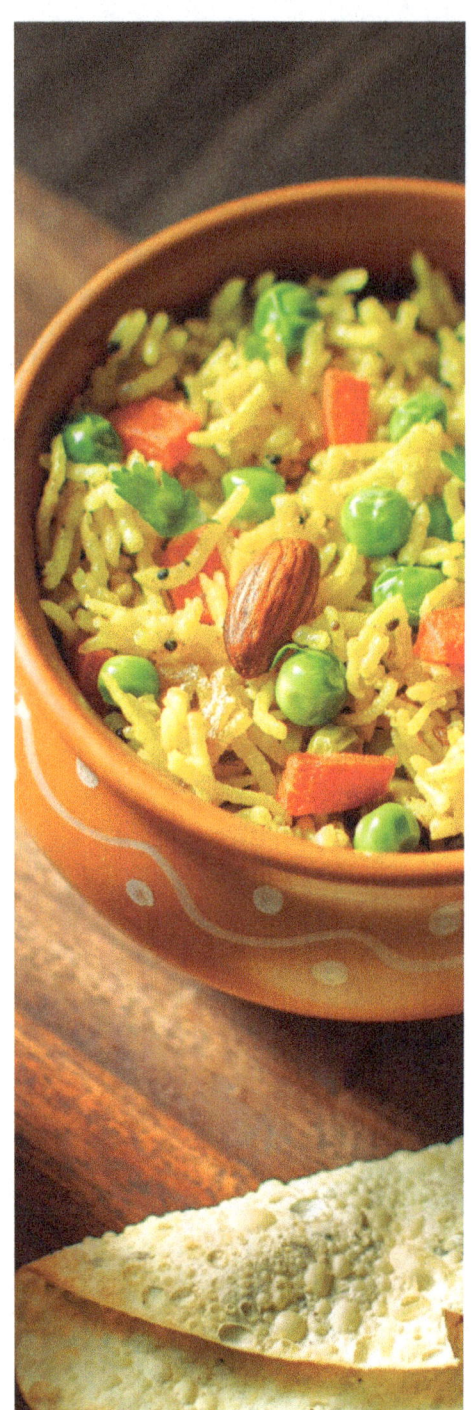

CARROT BIRYANI

Ingredients:
- 1 tablespoon olive oil
- 1 onion, diced
- 3 cloves garlic, minced
- 1 teaspoon ground turmeric
- 1 teaspoon ground cumin
- 1 teaspoon garam masala
- Salt and black pepper to taste
- 3 cups cooked basmati rice
- 2 cups grated carrots
- 1 cup frozen peas, thawed

Instructions:
1. Heat olive oil in a large pot over medium heat. Add onion, garlic, turmeric, cumin, garam masala, salt and black pepper. Cook until onions are translucent.
2. Stir in cooked rice, carrots, and peas. Mix well and cook for 5-7 minutes more, or until heated through. Serve immediately!

Serving Size: 1 bowl
Calories: 440

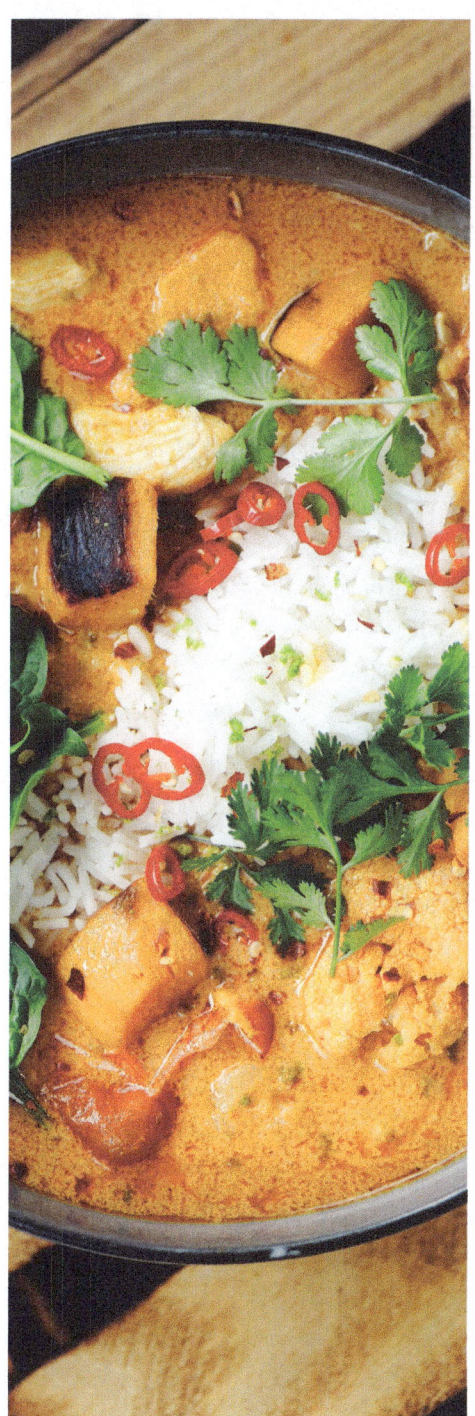

CURRIED COD WITH COCONUT RICE

Ingredients:
- 1 tablespoon olive oil
- 1 onion, diced
- 3 cloves garlic, minced
- 2 tablespoons curry powder
- Salt and black pepper to taste
- 4 cod filets (about 6 ounces each)
- 1 cup light coconut milk
- 2 cups cooked basmati rice
- 1/4 cup chopped cilantro

Instructions:
1. Heat olive oil in a large skillet over medium heat. Add onion, garlic, curry powder, salt and black pepper. Cook until onions are translucent.
2. Stir in cod filets and cook for 3-5 minutes per side, or until fish is cooked through.
3. Stir in coconut milk and cooked rice. Mix well and cook for 5-7 minutes more, or until heated through.
4. Serve immediately with cilantro on top!

Serving Size: 1 filet + 1 cup of rice
Calories: 610

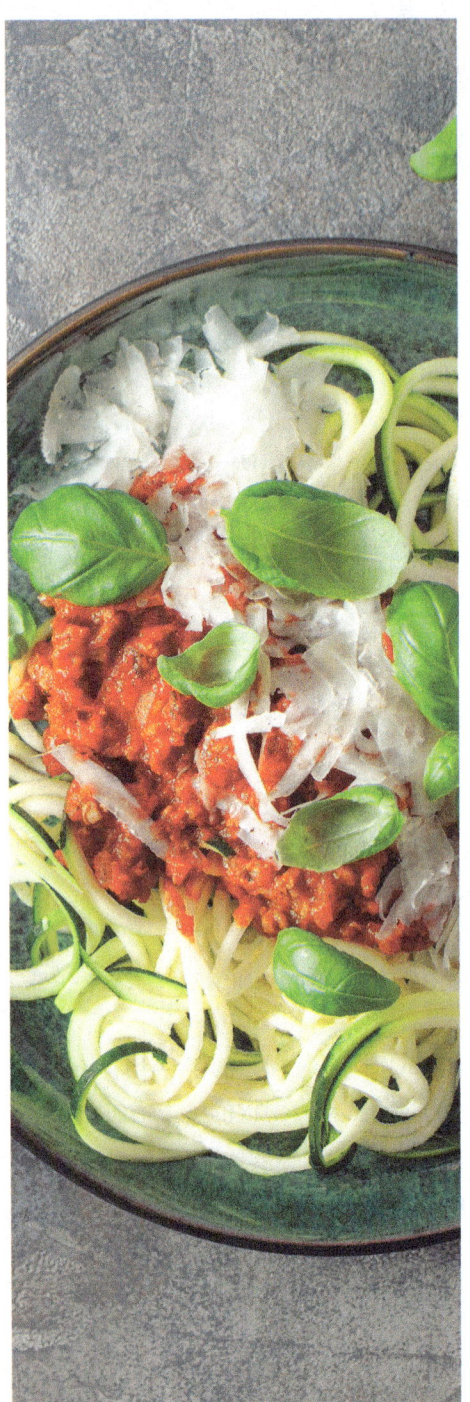

SEARED TILAPIA WITH SPIRALIZED ZUCCHINI

Ingredients:
- 1 tablespoon olive oil
- 4 tilapia filets (about 6 ounces each)
- Noodles/no fish (optional sub)
- Salt and black pepper to taste
- 2 tablespoons chopped parsley

For the zucchini noodles:
- 3 large zucchini, spiralized
- 1/4 teaspoon salt
- 1 tablespoon olive oil

Instructions:
1. Heat olive oil in a large skillet over medium-high heat. Add tilapia filets and season with salt and black pepper. Cook for 3-5 minutes per side, or until fish is cooked through. Remove from pan and set aside.
2. Add spiralized zucchini noodles to the same skillet and season with salt. Cook for 4-5 minutes, or until slightly softened.
3. Divide zucchini noodles among four plates and top with seared tilapia filets. Sprinkle with parsley and serve immediately!

Serving Size: 1 plate
Calories: 450

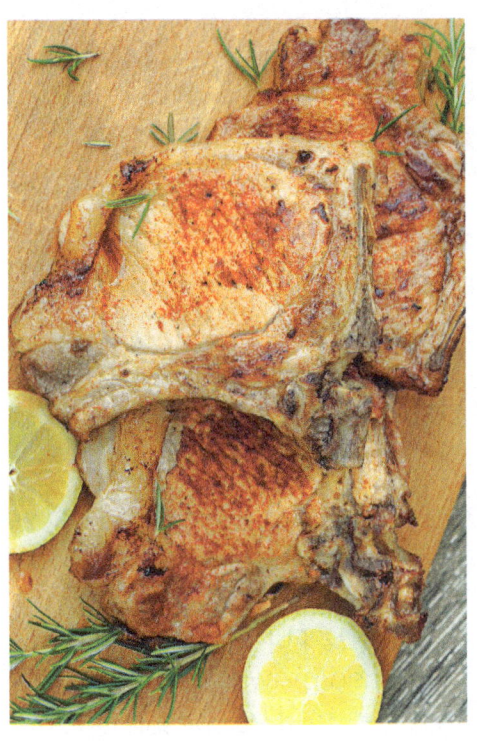

SHEET-PAN ITALIAN PORK CHOPS

Ingredients:
- 4 pork chops (about 6 ounces each)
- Salt and black pepper to taste
- 1 tablespoon olive oil
- 1/2 teaspoon dried basil
- 1/2 teaspoon dried oregano
- 1/4 teaspoon garlic powder

For the vegetables:
- 8-10 baby potatoes, halved
- 1 large onion, cut into wedges
- 1 red bell pepper, cut into chunks

Instructions:
1. Preheat oven to 425 degrees F.
2. Season pork chops with salt and black pepper. In a small bowl, mix together olive oil, basil, oregano, and garlic powder. Rub over pork chops.
3. Place pork chops on a greased baking sheet and bake for 15 minutes.
4. Meanwhile, mix together baby potatoes, onion wedges, and bell pepper chunks. Season with salt and black pepper.
5. Remove baking sheet from oven and add vegetables to the same sheet. Toss to coat with pan juices. Bake for 20-25 minutes more, or until vegetables are tender and pork chops are fully cooked. Serve immediately!

Serving Size: 1 pork chop
Calories: 520

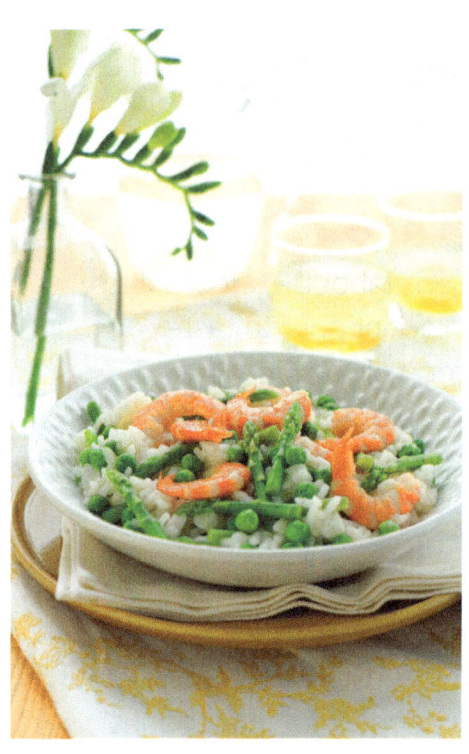

PRAWN, FENNEL, AND ASPARAGUS RISOTTO

Ingredients:
- 1 tablespoon olive oil
- 1/2 cup diced onion
- 3 cloves garlic, minced
- 1 fennel bulb, diced
- Salt and black pepper to taste
- 1 1/2 cups Arborio rice
- 4 cups chicken broth
- 1 bunch asparagus, cut into 1-inch pieces (about 1 1/2 cups)
- 1/2 pound cooked prawns
- 1/4 cup freshly grated Parmesan cheese

Instructions:
1. Heat olive oil in a large pot over medium heat. Add onion, garlic, and fennel. Season with salt and black pepper. Cook for 5-7 minutes, or until vegetables are softened.
2. Stir in Arborio rice and cook for 2 minutes more.
3. Slowly add chicken broth, 1 cup at a time, stirring constantly. Cook for 18-20 minutes, or until rice is tender and creamy.
4. Stir in asparagus pieces and cooked prawns. Cook for 3-5 minutes more, or until asparagus is slightly softened.
5. Remove from heat and stir in Parmesan cheese. Serve immediately!

Serving Size: 1 bowl
Calories: 630

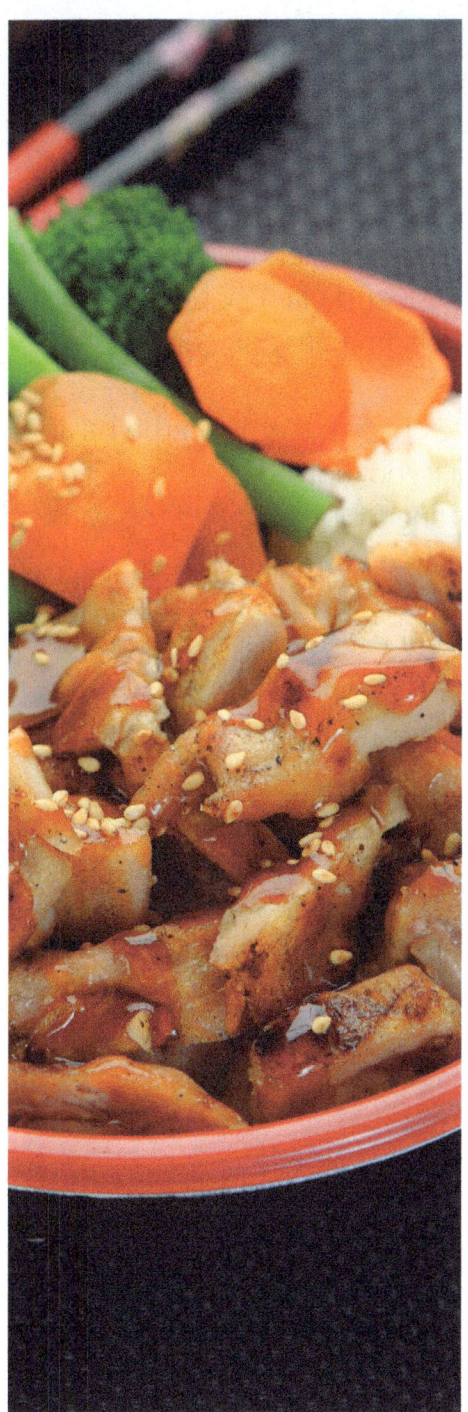

CHICKEN TERIYAKI BOWLS WITH CAULIFLOWER RICE

Ingredients:
- 1/2 cup soy sauce
- 1/2 cup honey
- 3 cloves garlic, minced
- 1 teaspoon ground ginger
- Salt and black pepper to taste
- 1 1/2 pounds boneless, skinless chicken thighs

For the cauliflower rice:
- 1 tablespoon olive oil
- 4 cups cauliflower florets
- Salt and black pepper to taste
- 3 green onions, thinly sliced

Instructions:

1. In a large bowl, whisk together soy sauce, honey, garlic, ginger, salt, and black pepper. Add chicken thighs and toss to coat. Let marinate for at least 30 minutes (up to 8 hours).
2. Preheat oven to 375 degrees F.
3. To make the cauliflower rice, heat olive oil in a large skillet over medium-high heat. Add cauliflower florets and season with salt and black pepper. Cook for 5-7 minutes, or until slightly softened. Remove from heat and stir in green onions.
4. Spray a baking sheet with cooking spray. Place chicken thighs on the baking sheet and bake for 25-30 minutes, or until fully cooked.
5. To assemble bowls, divide cauliflower rice among four bowls and top with chicken thighs and any remaining marinade. Serve immediately!

Serving Size: 1 bowl
Calories: 520

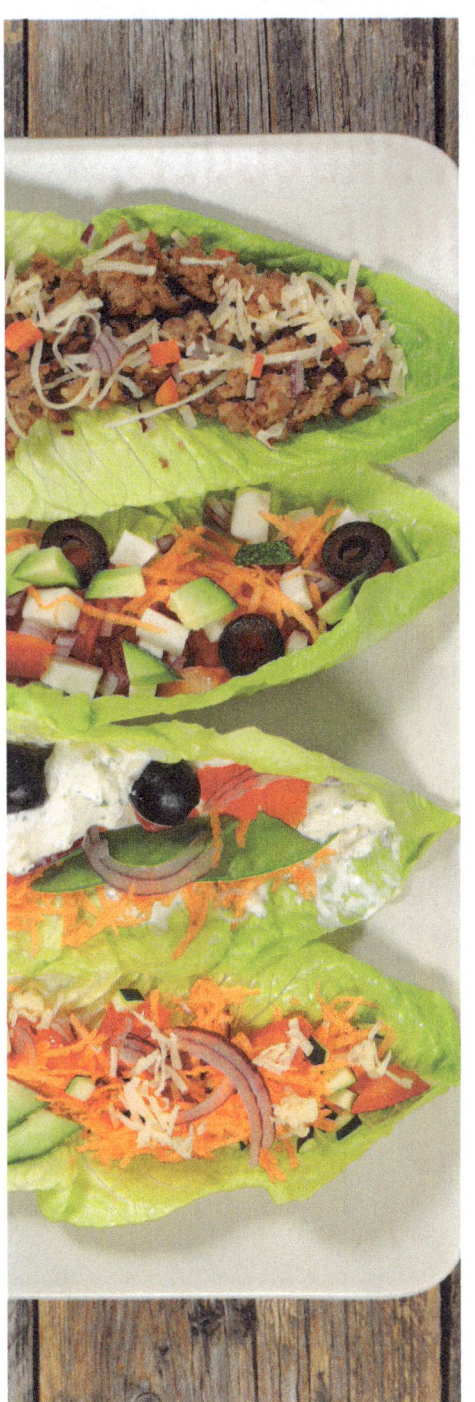

TEMPEH LETTUCE WRAPS

Ingredients:
- 8 ounces tempeh, diced
- 1 tablespoon olive oil
- 3 cloves garlic, minced
- 1/2 teaspoon ground ginger
- Salt and black pepper to taste
- 1/4 cup hoisin sauce
- 2 tablespoons rice vinegar
- 1 tablespoon Sriracha sauce
- 1 head iceberg lettuce, leaves separated

Instructions:
1. Heat olive oil in a large skillet over medium heat. Add tempeh, garlic, and ginger. Season with salt and black pepper. Cook for 5-7 minutes, or until slightly browned.
2. In a small bowl, whisk together hoisin sauce, rice vinegar, and Sriracha sauce. Add to the tempeh mixture and cook for 2-3 minutes, or until heated through.
3. Spoon mixture into lettuce leaves and serve immediately!

Serving Size: 2 wraps
Calories: 190

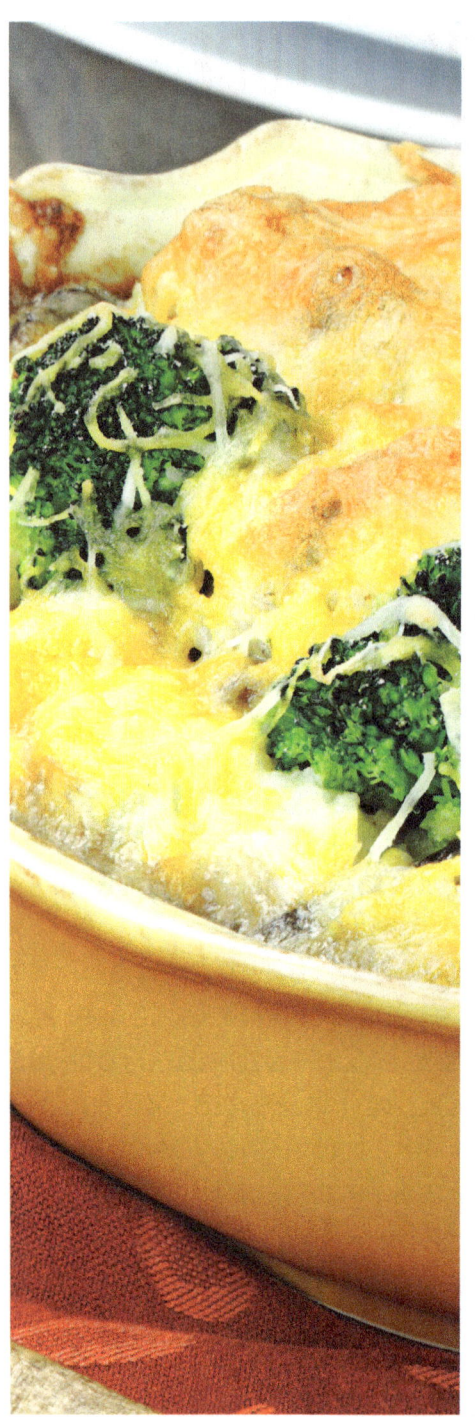

CREAMY CHICKEN QUINOA BROCCOLI CASSEROLE

Ingredients:

- 1 tablespoon olive oil
- 1 onion, diced
- 3 cloves garlic, minced
- Salt and black pepper to taste
- 1 pound boneless, skinless chicken breasts, cut into 1-inch cubes
- 1/2 cup quinoa, rinsed and drained
- 1 head broccoli, cut into florets (about 3 cups)

For the sauce:

- 1/4 cup all-purpose flour
- 1 cup chicken broth
- 1 cup milk

Instructions:
1. Preheat oven to 375 degrees F.
2. Heat olive oil in a large pot over medium heat. Add onion, garlic, salt, and black pepper. Cook for 5-7 minutes, or until softened.
3. Stir in chicken and cook for 5 minutes more.
4. Stir in quinoa and broccoli and cook for 2 minutes more.
5. To make the sauce, whisk together flour, chicken broth, and milk in a small bowl. Pour over the casserole and stir to combine.
6. 6Bake for 20-25 minutes, or until bubbly and golden brown on top. Serve immediately!

Serving Size: 1/6 of casserole
Calories: 380

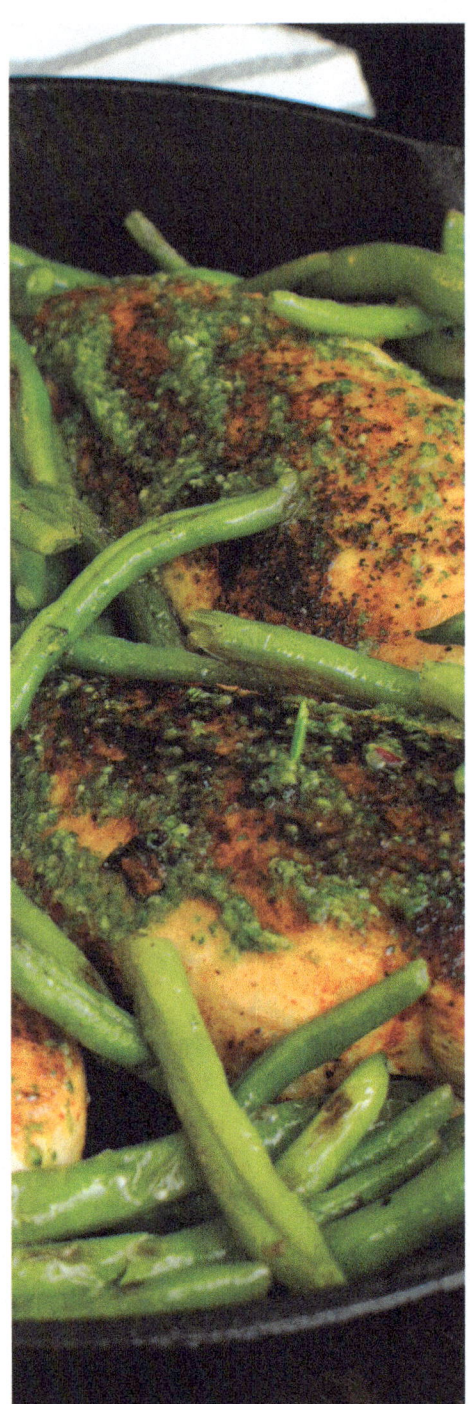

SIMPLE SESAME CHICKEN WITH GREEN BEANS

Ingredients:
- 1 tablespoon olive oil
- 1 onion, diced
- 3 cloves garlic, minced
- Salt and black pepper to taste
- 1 pound boneless, skinless chicken breasts, cut into 1-inch cubes
- 1/4 cup all-purpose flour
- 2 tablespoons sesame seeds
- 1 cup chicken broth
- 1/4 cup honey
- 2 tablespoons rice vinegar

For the green beans:
- 1 tablespoon olive oil
- 1 pound green beans, trimmed and cut into 1-inch pieces

Instructions:

1. Heat olive oil in a large skillet over medium heat. Add onion, garlic, salt, and black pepper. Cook for 5-7 minutes, or until softened.
2. Stir in chicken and cook for 5 minutes more.
3. Sprinkle flour and sesame seeds over the chicken and stir to combine.
4. Pour in chicken broth, honey, and rice vinegar. Stir to combine and bring to a simmer. Let cook for 2-3 minutes, or until slightly thickened.
5. Meanwhile, heat olive oil in a separate skillet over medium-high heat. Add green beans and cook for 5-7 minutes, or until slightly softened.
6. Serve chicken and sauce over green beans and enjoy!

Serving Size: 1/4 of recipe
Calories: 420

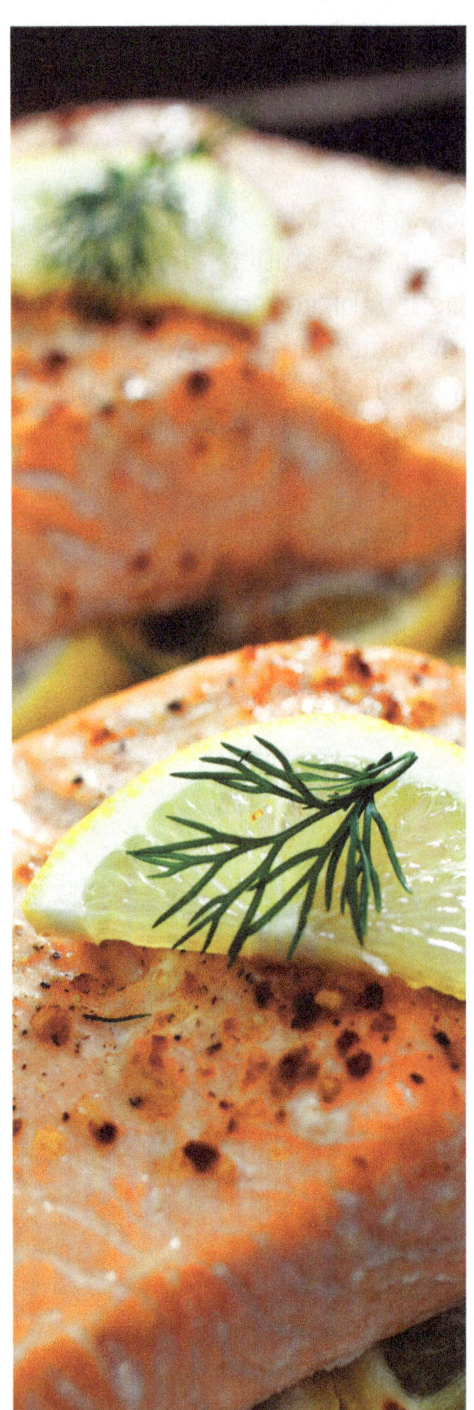

HARISSA AND CITRUS BAKED SALMON

Ingredients:
- 4 (6-ounce) salmon filets
- Salt and black pepper to taste
- 1/2 teaspoon cumin
- 1 tablespoon olive oil
- 1/4 cup harissa paste
- Juice of 1 lemon
- Zest of 1 lemon

Instructions:
1. Preheat oven to 400 degrees F.
2. Season salmon filets with salt, black pepper, and cumin. Heat olive oil in a large skillet over medium-high heat. Add salmon filets and cook for 3-4 minutes per side, or until browned.
3. In a small bowl, whisk together harissa paste, lemon juice, and lemon zest. Spread over the top of the salmon filets.
4. Bake for 12-15 minutes, or until cooked through. Serve immediately!

Serving Size: 1 salmon filet
Calories: 290

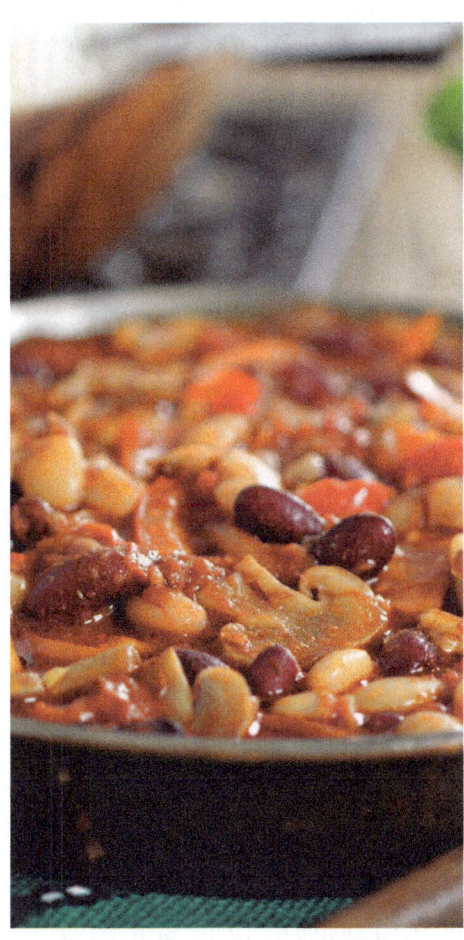

VEGAN CHILI

Ingredients:

- 1 tablespoon olive oil
- 1 onion, diced
- 3 cloves garlic, minced
- Salt and black pepper to taste
- 1 pound Impossible beef
- 2 tablespoons chili powder
- 1 teaspoon cumin
- 1 teaspoon smoked paprika
- 1 teaspoon oregano
- 1/2 teaspoon salt
- One 14.5-ounce can diced tomatoes, undrained
- One 15-ounce can kidney beans, drained and rinsed
- One 15-ounce can black beans, drained and rinsed
- One 8-ounce can tomato sauce

Instructions:

1. Heat olive oil in a large pot over medium heat. Add onion, garlic, salt, and black pepper. Cook for 5 minutes, or until softened.
2. Add Impossible beef and cook for 5 minutes more, or until browned.
3. Stir in chili powder, cumin, smoked paprika, oregano, and salt. Cook for 1 minute more.
4. Stir in diced tomatoes, kidney beans, black beans, and tomato sauce. Bring to a simmer and let cook for 10 minutes. Serve immediately!

Serving Size: 1/6 of recipe
Calories: 340

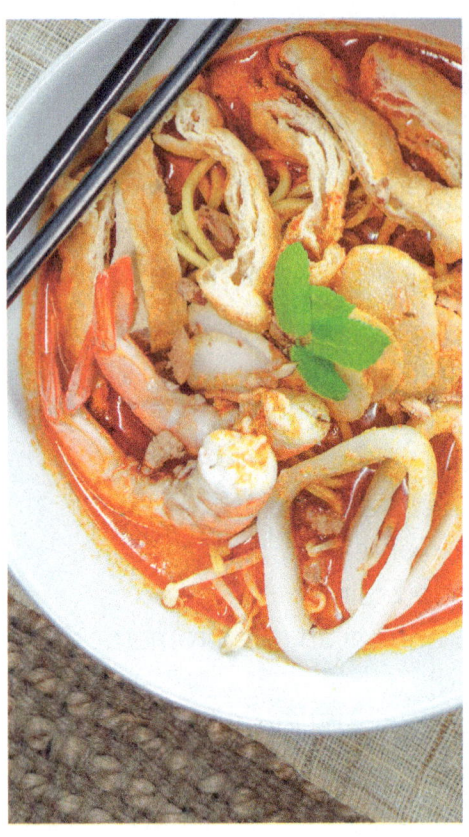

RICH PAPRIKA SEAFOOD BOWL

Ingredients:
- 1 tablespoon olive oil
- 1 onion, diced
- 3 cloves garlic, minced
- Salt and black pepper to taste
- 2 tablespoons paprika
- 1 teaspoon smoked paprika
- 1/4 teaspoon cayenne pepper
- 1 pound shrimp, peeled and deveined
- 8 ounces scallops
- 8 ounces cod filets, cut into 1-inch cubes
- One 14.5-ounce can diced tomatoes, undrained
- One 8-ounce can tomato sauce

Instructions:
1. Heat olive oil in a large pot over medium heat. Add onion, garlic, salt, and black pepper. Cook for 5 minutes, or until softened.
2. Stir in paprika, smoked paprika, and cayenne pepper. Cook for 1 minute more.
3. Add shrimp, scallops, and cod. Cook for 3-5 minutes, or until cod is opaque and shrimp is pink.
4. Stir in diced tomatoes and tomato sauce. Bring to a simmer and let cook for 5 minutes. Serve immediately!

Serving Size: 1 bowl
Calories: 380

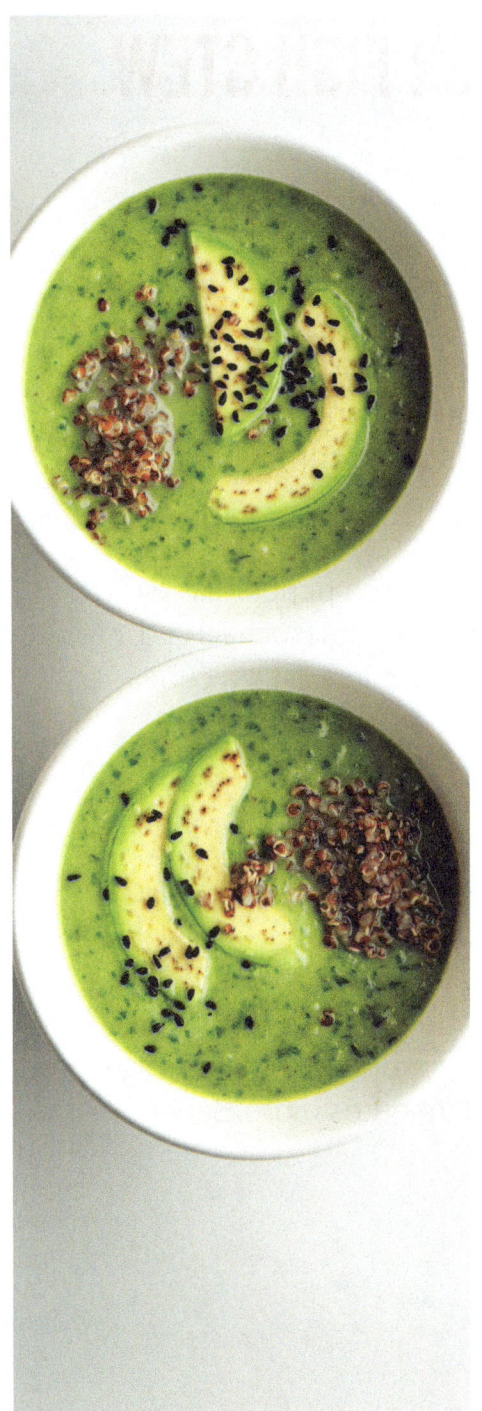

AVOCADO SOUP

Ingredients:
- 3 avocados, peeled and pitted
- 1/2 lime, juiced
- 1/2 cup cilantro leaves
- 1 jalapeno, seeded and diced
- 1 tablespoon olive oil
- Salt and black pepper to taste
- 4 cups chicken or vegetable broth

Instructions:
1. Add avocados, lime juice, cilantro, jalapeno, olive oil, salt, and black pepper to a blender. Blend until smooth.
2. Pour avocado mixture into a large pot over medium heat. Stir in chicken broth. Bring to a simmer and let cook for 5 minutes. Serve immediately!

Serving Size: 1 bowl
Calories: 280

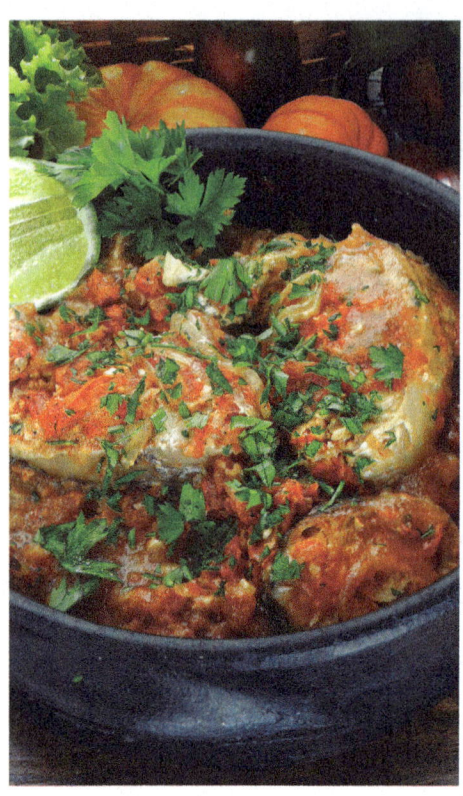

SUMMER FISH STEW

Ingredients:

- 1 tablespoon olive oil
- 1 onion, diced
- 3 cloves garlic, minced
- Salt and black pepper to taste
- 2 tablespoons tomato paste
- One 28-ounce can crushed tomatoes
- One 8-ounce can tomato sauce
- 1/4 cup white wine
- 1 teaspoon oregano
- 1/4 teaspoon red pepper flakes
- 2 pounds fish filets (such as cod, halibut, or salmon), cut into 1-inch cubes
- 1 zucchini, diced
- 1 yellow squash, diced

Instructions:

1. Heat olive oil in a large pot over medium heat. Add onion, garlic, salt, and black pepper. Cook for 5 minutes, or until softened.
2. Stir in tomato paste, crushed tomatoes, tomato sauce, white wine, oregano, and red pepper flakes. Bring to a simmer and let cook for 10 minutes.
3. Stir in fish cubes and let cook for 3-5 minutes, or until cooked through. Add zucchini and yellow squash and let cook for 5 minutes more. Serve immediately!

Serving Size: 1 bowl
Calories: 400

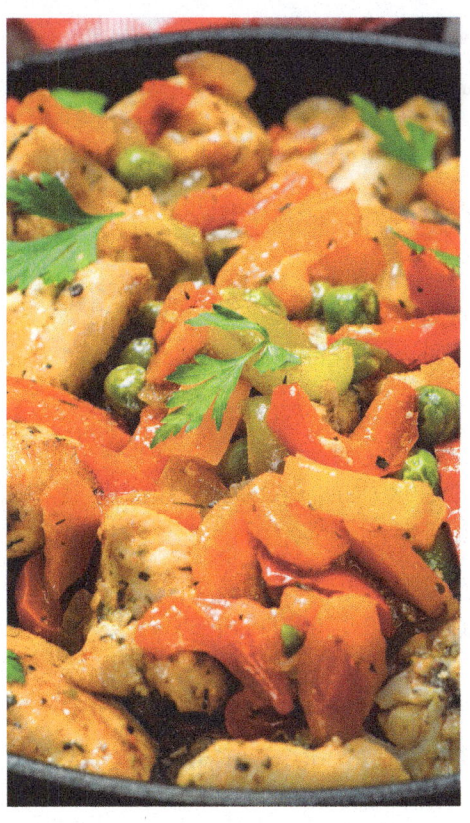

ONE SKILLET LEMON CHICKEN AND BELL PEPPERS AND SPINACH

Ingredients:

- 1 tablespoon olive oil
- 1 onion, diced
- 3 cloves garlic, minced
- Salt and black pepper to taste
- 1 pound boneless, skinless chicken breasts, cut into 1-inch cubes
- 1 red bell pepper, diced
- 1 green bell pepper, diced
- 4 cups baby spinach leaves
- 1/4 cup chicken broth
- 2 tablespoons lemon juice

Instructions:

1. Heat olive oil in a large skillet over medium heat. Add onion, garlic, salt, and black pepper. Cook for 5 minutes, or until softened.
2. Stir in chicken cubes and cook for 5 minutes more, or until browned.
3. Add bell peppers and cook for 3-5 minutes, or until softened.
4. Stir in baby spinach leaves and chicken broth and let cook for 2 minutes, or until spinach is wilted. Finally, stir in lemon juice. Serve immediately!

Serving Size: 1/6 of recipe
Calories: 310

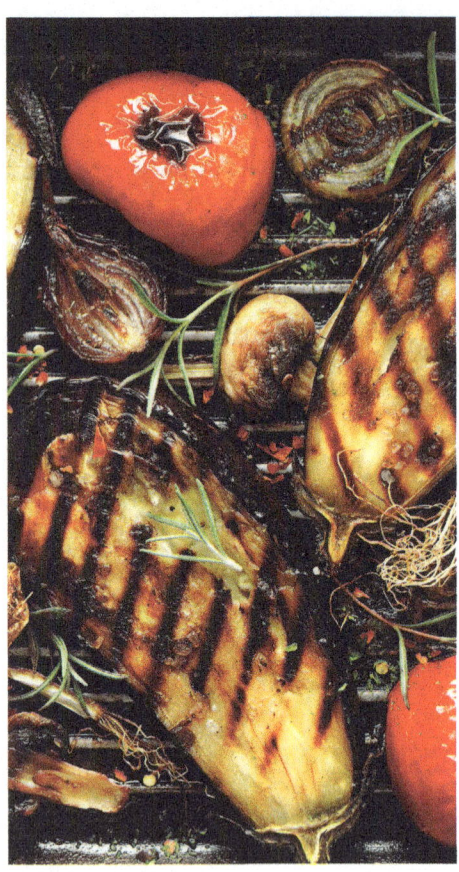

SPICED GRILLED EGGPLANT WITH FRESH TOMATO SALAD

Ingredients:
- 1 large eggplant, sliced into 1-inch rounds
- Olive oil spray
- Salt and black pepper to taste
- 1 teaspoon chili powder
- 1 teaspoon cumin
- 1/4 cup chopped fresh parsley
- 1/4 cup chopped fresh mint
- 3 tablespoons olive oil, divided
- 2 cups cherry tomatoes, halved
- 1/2 red onion, diced
- Juice of 1 lemon

Instructions:
1. Preheat grill to medium-high heat.
2. Spray eggplant rounds with olive oil and season with salt, black pepper, chili powder, and cumin. Grill for 5-7 minutes per side, or until tender.
3. In a small bowl, mix together parsley, mint, 2 tablespoons olive oil, cherry tomatoes, red onion, and lemon juice. Season with salt and black pepper to taste.
4. Serve grilled eggplant rounds topped with fresh tomato salad.

Serving Size: 1/6 of recipe
Calories: 210

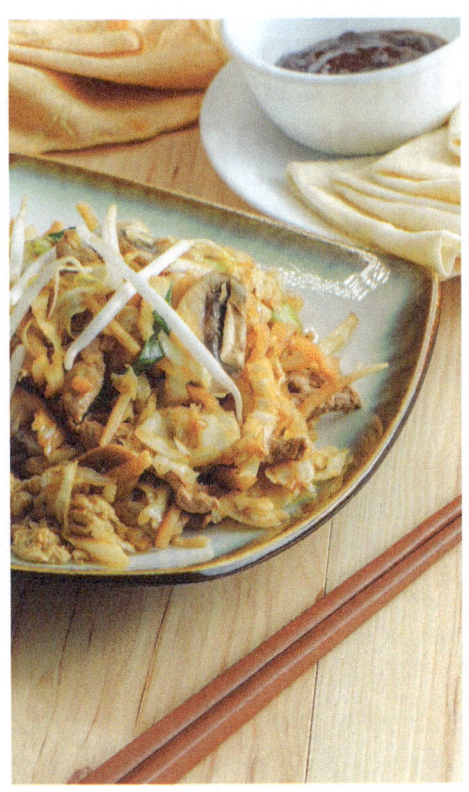

MOO SHU MUSHROOM WRAPS

Ingredients:

- 8 ounces mushrooms, diced
- 1/4 cup water
- 2 tablespoons soy sauce
- 1 tablespoon rice vinegar
- 1 teaspoon sugar
- 1/2 teaspoon sesame oil
- 3 cloves garlic, minced
- 1-inch piece ginger, peeled and grated
- Salt and black pepper to taste
- 6 whole wheat tortillas
- 1/4 cup hoisin sauce
- 2 cups shredded cabbage mix

Instructions:

1. In a large skillet over medium heat, add mushrooms, water, soy sauce, rice vinegar, sugar, sesame oil, garlic, ginger, salt, and black pepper. Cook for 5 minutes.
2. Add cabbage mix and cook for 3-5 minutes more, or until wilted.
3. Warm tortillas in the microwave for 30 seconds. Spread each one with hoisin sauce, and then top with mushroom mixture. Roll up and serve immediately!

Serving Size: 1 wrap
Calories: 260

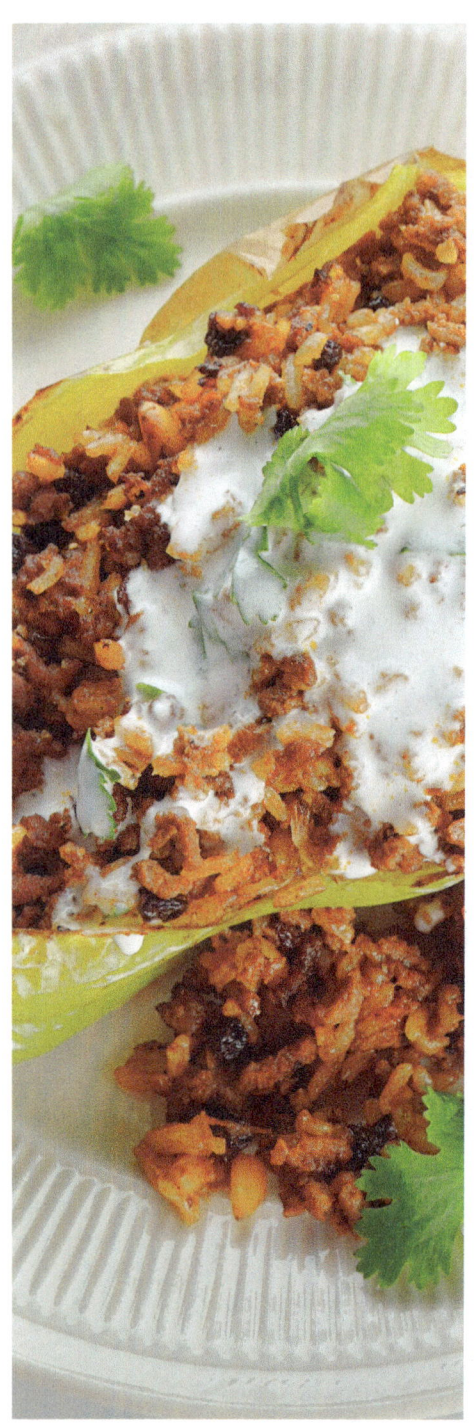

CHILI-STUFFED POBLANO PEPPERS

Ingredients:

- 4 large poblano peppers
- 1 tablespoon olive oil
- 1 onion, diced
- 3 cloves garlic, minced
- Salt and black pepper to taste
- 1 pound lean ground beef
- 1 tablespoon chili powder
- 2 teaspoons cumin
- One 14.5-ounce can diced tomatoes, drained
- One 15-ounce can black beans, rinsed and drained
- 1/2 cup prepared salsa
- 1/2 cup shredded cheddar cheese

Instructions:

1. Preheat oven to 350 degrees F.
2. Cut a slit down the middle of each poblano pepper. In a large skillet over medium heat, add olive oil, onion, garlic, salt, and black pepper. Cook for 5 minutes, or until softened.
3. Add ground beef and cook for 5 minutes more, or until browned. Stir in chili powder and cumin.
4. Stir in diced tomatoes, black beans, salsa, and cheddar cheese. Let mixture cool for 5 minutes.
5. Spoon mixture into poblano peppers and place on a baking sheet. Bake for 20-25 minutes, or until peppers are tender. Serve immediately!

Serving Size: 1 pepper
Calories: 310

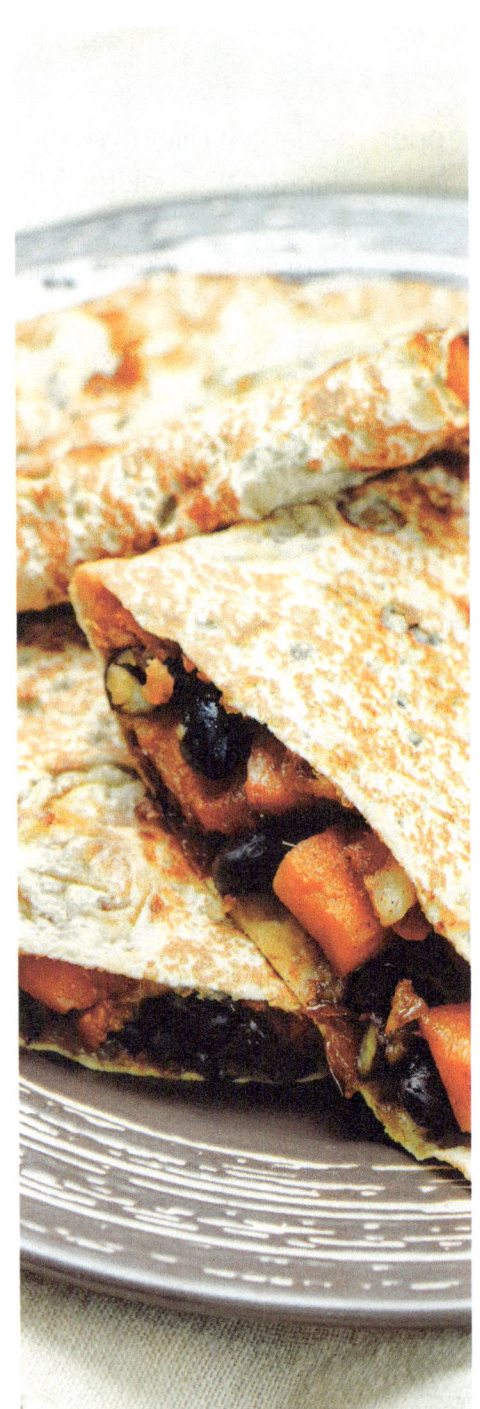

SWEET POTATO & BEAN QUESADILLAS

Ingredients:
- 1 large sweet potato, peeled and grated
- One 15-ounce can black beans, rinsed and drained
- 1/4 cup prepared salsa
- 1 teaspoon chili powder
- Salt and black pepper to taste
- 4 whole wheat tortillas
- 1/2 cup shredded cheddar cheeses

Instructions:
1. Preheat oven to 350 degrees F.
2. In a large bowl, mix together sweet potato, black beans, salsa, chili powder, salt, and black pepper.
3. Place 2 tortillas on a baking sheet. Top each one with sweet potato mixture and cheddar cheese. Top with remaining tortillas.
4. Bake for 20-25 minutes, or until tortillas are crispy. Cut each quesadilla into 4 pieces and serve immediately!

Serving Size: 1 quesadilla
Calories: 260

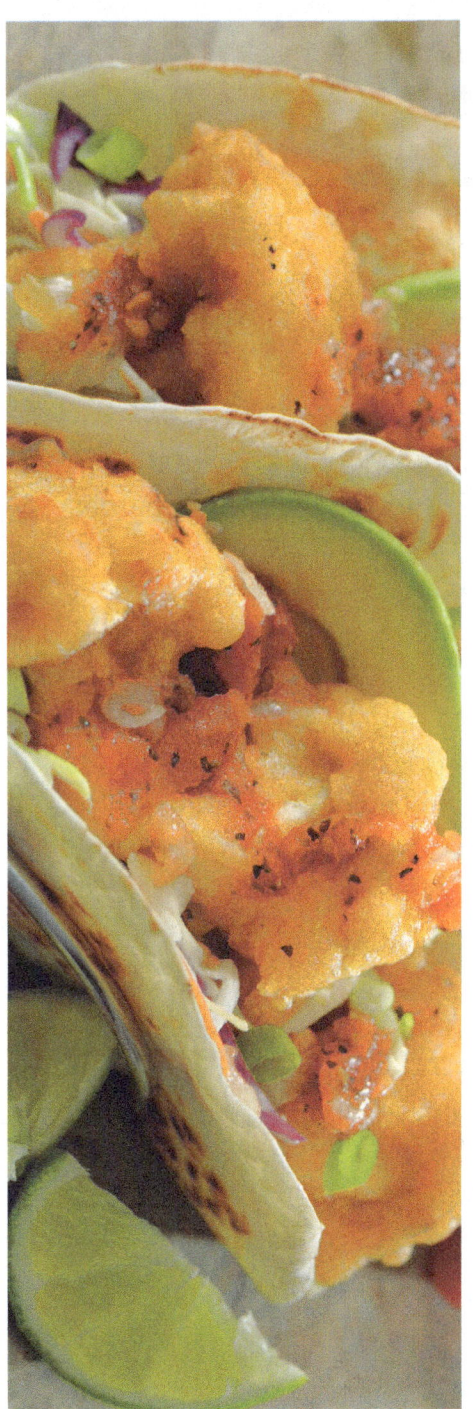

ROASTED CAULIFLOWER TACOS WITH CHIPOTLE CREAM

Ingredients:
- 1 head cauliflower, cut into florets
- Olive oil spray
- Salt and black pepper to taste
- 1/2 cup prepared salsa
- 1/4 cup plain Greek yogurt
- 1 tablespoon adobo sauce
- 1 teaspoon chili powder
- 6 whole wheat tortillas

Instructions:
1. Preheat oven to 400 degrees F.
2. Line a baking sheet with parchment paper and spray with olive oil. Add cauliflower florets and season with salt, black pepper, and chili powder. Roast for 25 minutes, or until tender.
3. In a small bowl, mix together salsa, Greek yogurt, adobo sauce, and chili powder.
4. Warm tortillas in the microwave for 30 seconds. Assemble tacos by adding roasted cauliflower and chipotle cream sauce to each tortilla. Serve immediately!

Serving Size: 1 taco
Calories: 210

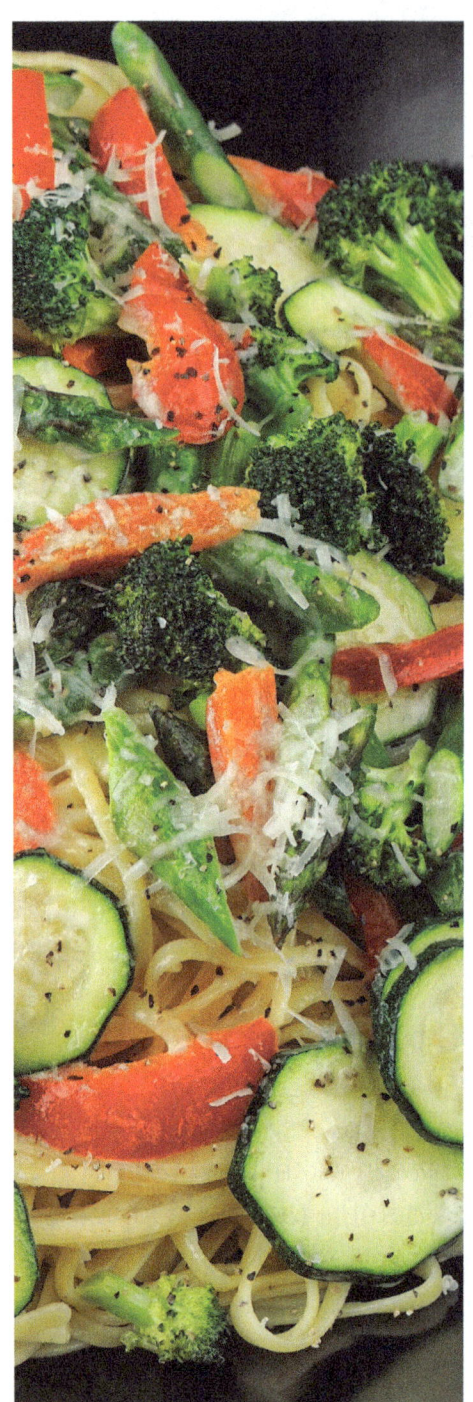

BROCCOLI VEGGIE PASTA PRIMAVERA

Ingredients:

- 1 tablespoon olive oil
- 3 cloves garlic, minced
- 1 onion, diced
- Salt and black pepper to taste
- 2 heads broccoli, cut into florets
- One 14.5-ounce can diced tomatoes, drained
- 1/4 cup prepared pesto
- 8 ounces whole wheat pasta shells

Instructions:

1. In a large pot over medium heat, add olive oil, garlic, onion, salt, and black pepper. Cook for 5 minutes, or until softened.
2. Add broccoli and cook for 3 minutes more.
3. Stir in diced tomatoes and pesto. Add pasta shells and cook according to package instructions. Serve immediately!

Serving Size: 1 plate
Calories: 430

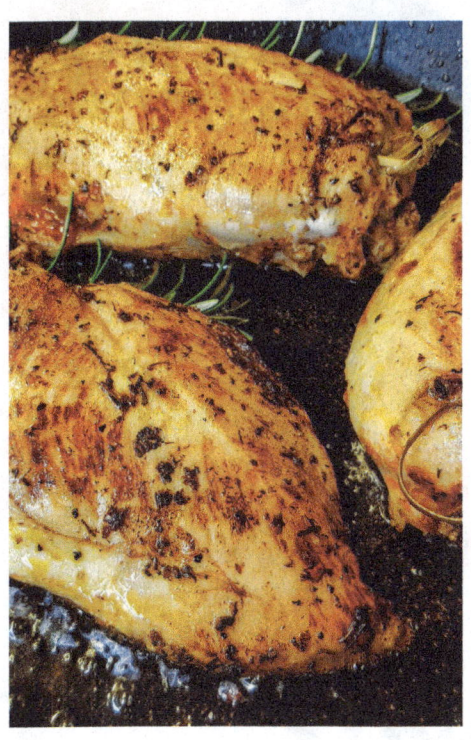

SEARED COCONUT LIME CHICKEN WITH SNAP PEA SLAW

Ingredients:

- 1 tablespoon olive oil
- 4 boneless, skinless chicken breasts
- Salt and black pepper to taste
- 1 teaspoon chili powder
- 1/2 teaspoon cumin
- 1 cup unsweetened coconut milk
- Juice of 2 limes
- 4 cups coleslaw mix
- 1/2 cup chopped fresh cilantro

Instructions:

1. In a large skillet over medium heat, add olive oil, chicken breasts, salt, black pepper, chili powder, and cumin. Cook for 5 minutes per side, or until browned.
2. Add coconut milk and lime juice to the pan and cook for 3 minutes more.
3. Remove chicken from the pan and let rest on a cutting board. Add coleslaw mix to the pan and cook for 3 minutes, or until tender.
4. Slice chicken into thin strips and add back to the pan. Stir in cilantro and serve immediately!

Serving Size: 1 plate
Calories: 510

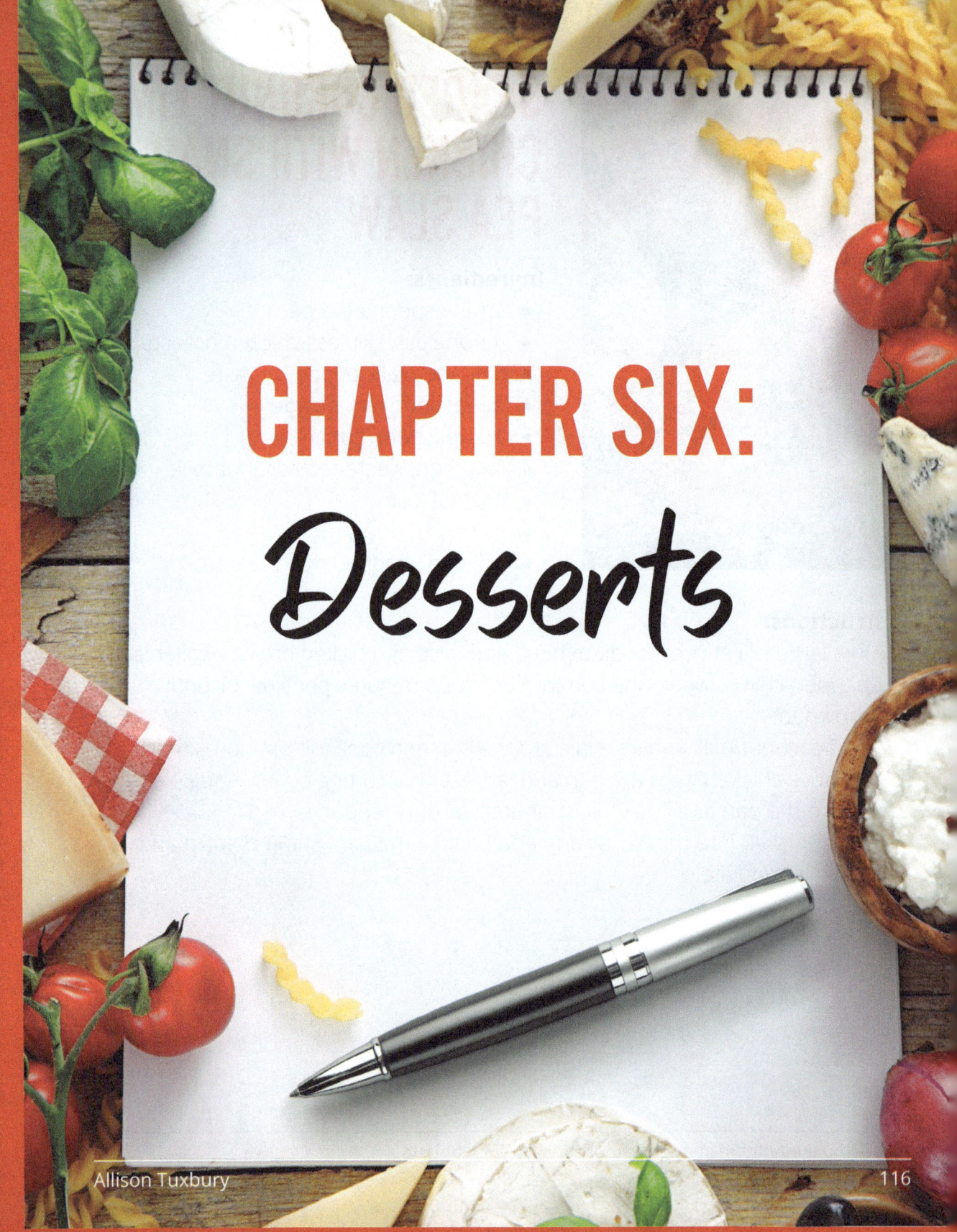

CHAPTER SIX:
Desserts

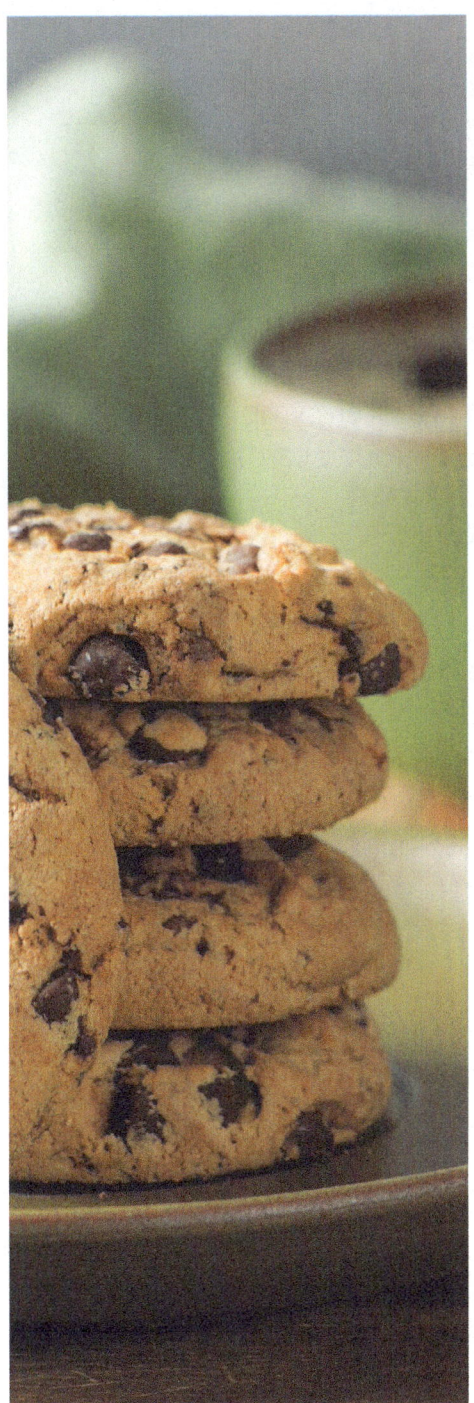

CHOCOLATE CHIP COOKIES

Ingredients:
- 1 cup almond butter
- 1/2 cup coconut sugar
- 1 egg
- 1 teaspoon baking soda
- 1/4 teaspoon salt
- 1 teaspoon vanilla extract
- 1 cup gluten-free flour
- 1/2 cup sugar-free chocolate chips

Instructions:
1. Preheat oven to 350 degrees F.
2. In a large bowl, mix together almond butter, coconut sugar, egg, baking soda, salt, and vanilla extract.
3. Stir in flour and chocolate chips until well combined.
4. Drop dough by the tablespoon onto a greased or lined baking sheet and press down slightly. Bake for 10-12 minutes, or until cookies are golden brown. Let cool on baking sheet for 5 minutes before transferring to a wire rack to cool completely.

Serving Size: 1 cookie
Calories: 140

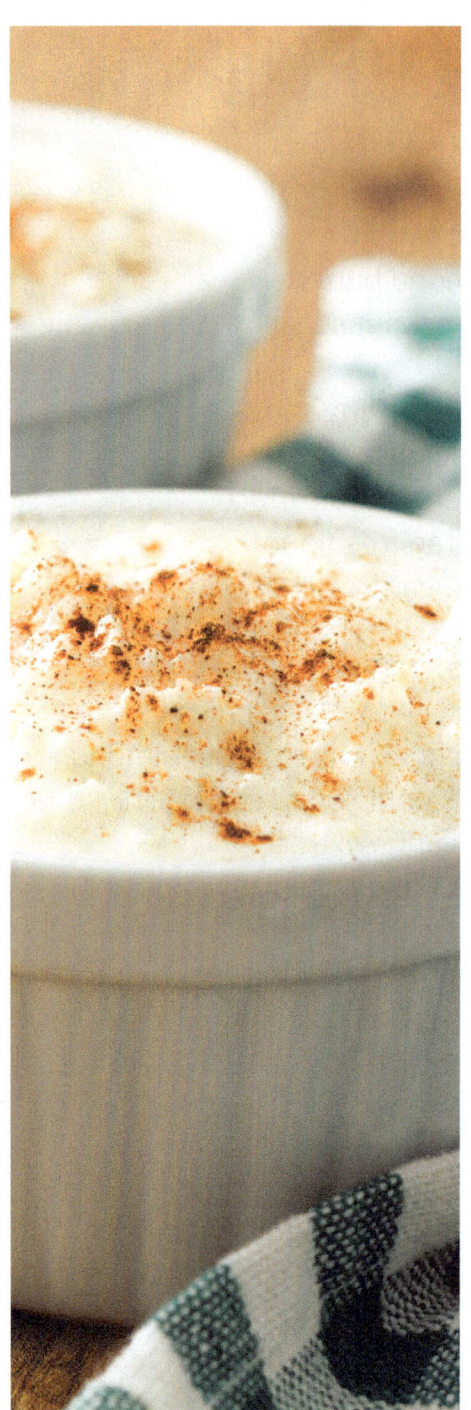

LEBANESE RICE PUDDING

Ingredients:

- 1 cup brown rice
- 2 cups water
- 1 (14-ounce) can full-fat coconut milk
- 1/2 cup sugar-free syrup
- 1 teaspoon ground cardamom

Instructions:

1. In a medium saucepan, bring rice and water to a boil. Lower heat and simmer for 15 minutes, or until fully cooked.
2. Add coconut milk, sugar-free syrup, and cardamom. Stir until well combined.
3. Raise heat to medium and cook for an additional 5 minutes, or until pudding has thickened. Serve immediately!

Serving Size: 1/2 cup
Calories: 210

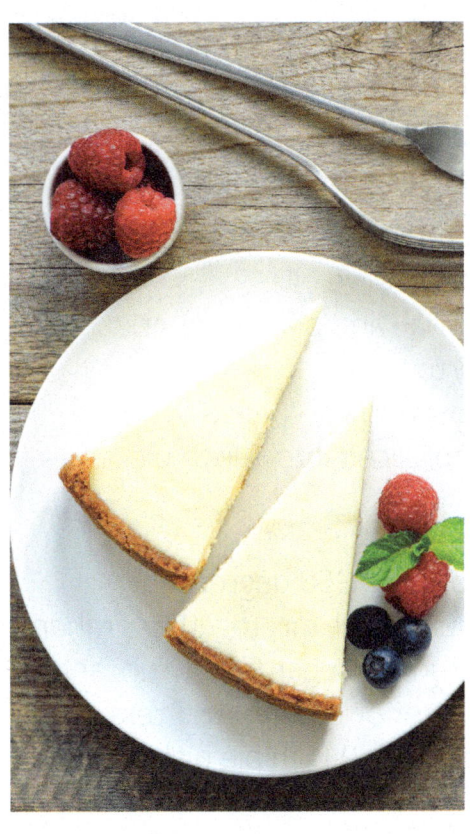

NEW YORK CHEESECAKE

Ingredients:
- For the crust:
-
- 1 1/2 cups graham cracker crumbs
- 3 tablespoons sugar-free syrup
- 6 tablespoons melted butter or margarine

For the filling:
- 4 (8-ounce) packages cream cheese, softened
- 1 cup sugar-free syrup
- 4 eggs
- 1 teaspoon vanilla extract

Instructions:
1. Preheat oven to 350 degrees F.
2. In a medium bowl, mix together graham cracker crumbs, sugar-free syrup, and melted butter or margarine. Press into the bottom of a 9-inch springform pan. Set aside.
3. In a large bowl, beat cream cheese until smooth. Beat in sugar-free syrup, eggs, and vanilla extract until well combined. Pour over crust.
4. Bake for 45-50 minutes, or until cheesecake is firm. Let cool completely before serving.

Serving Size: 1 slice
Calories: 420

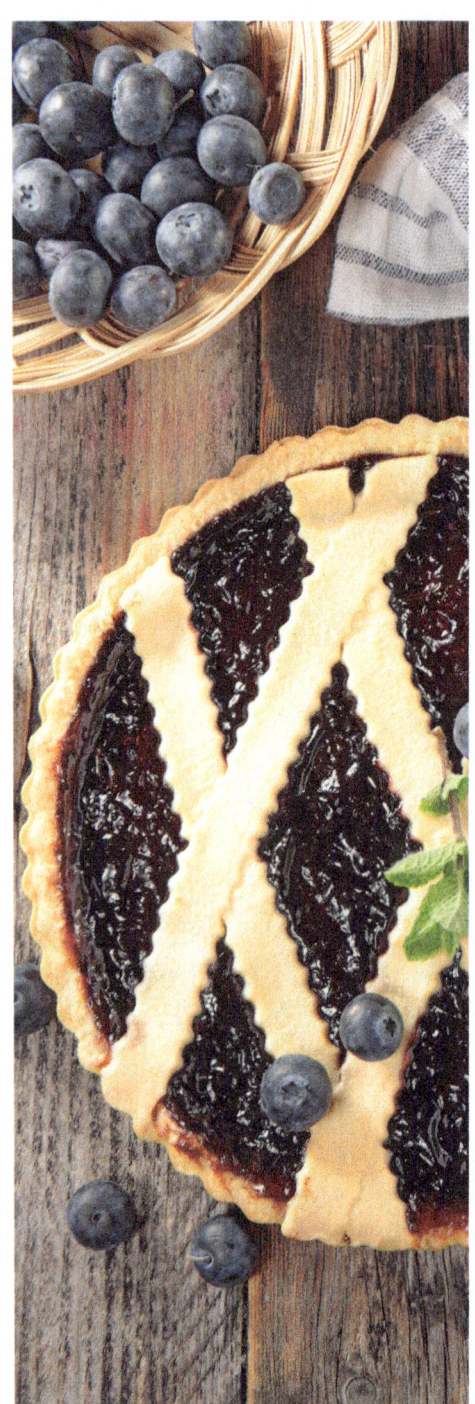

BLUEBERRY PIE

Ingredients:

- 1 cup diced tomatoes
- 1/4 cup chopped fresh basil
- 1 tablespoon olive oil
- Salt (optional) and black pepper (optional) to taste
- 1 ball (8 oz) burrata cheese
- 1 baguette, sliced into 1-inch pieces

Instructions:

1. Preheat oven to 350 degrees F.
2. In a medium bowl, mix together graham cracker crumbs, sugar-free syrup, and melted butter or margarine. Press into the bottom of a 9-inch pie dish. Set aside.
3. In a large bowl, mix together blueberries, sugar-free syrup, and cornstarch or tapioca flour. Pour into crust.
4. Bake for 45-50 minutes, or until filling is bubbly and crust is golden brown. Let cool completely before serving.

Serving Size: 1 slice
Calories: 340

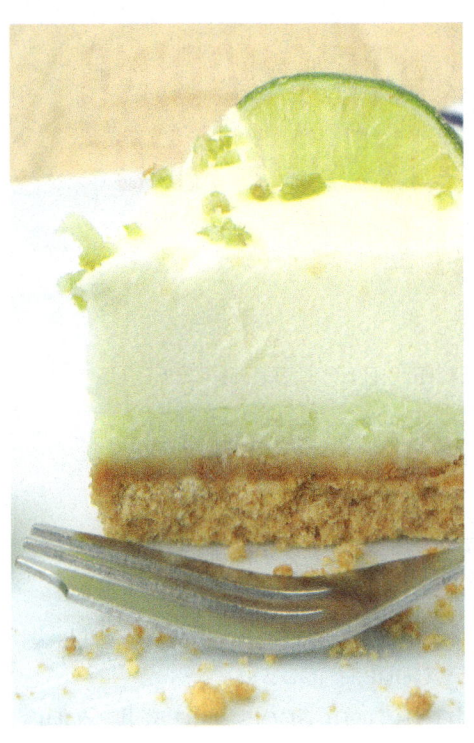

LOW-FAT SUGAR-FREE KEY LIME PIE

Ingredients:

For the crust:
- 1 1/2 cups graham cracker crumbs
- 3 tablespoons sugar-free syrup
- 6 tablespoons melted butter or margarine

For the filling:
- 2 (14-ounce) cans low-fat coconut milk
- 1/2 cup sugar-free limeade concentrate
- 3 tablespoons cornstarch or tapioca flour

Instructions:

1. Preheat oven to 350 degrees F.
2. In a medium bowl, mix together graham cracker crumbs, sugar-free syrup, and melted butter or margarine. Press into the bottom of a 9-inch pie dish. Set aside.
3. In a large saucepan, whisk together coconut milk, sugar-free limeade concentrate, and cornstarch or tapioca flour. Cook over medium heat, stirring constantly, until mixture comes to a boil.
4. Pour into crust and bake for 15 minutes. Let cool completely before serving.

Serving Size: 1 slice
Calories: 330

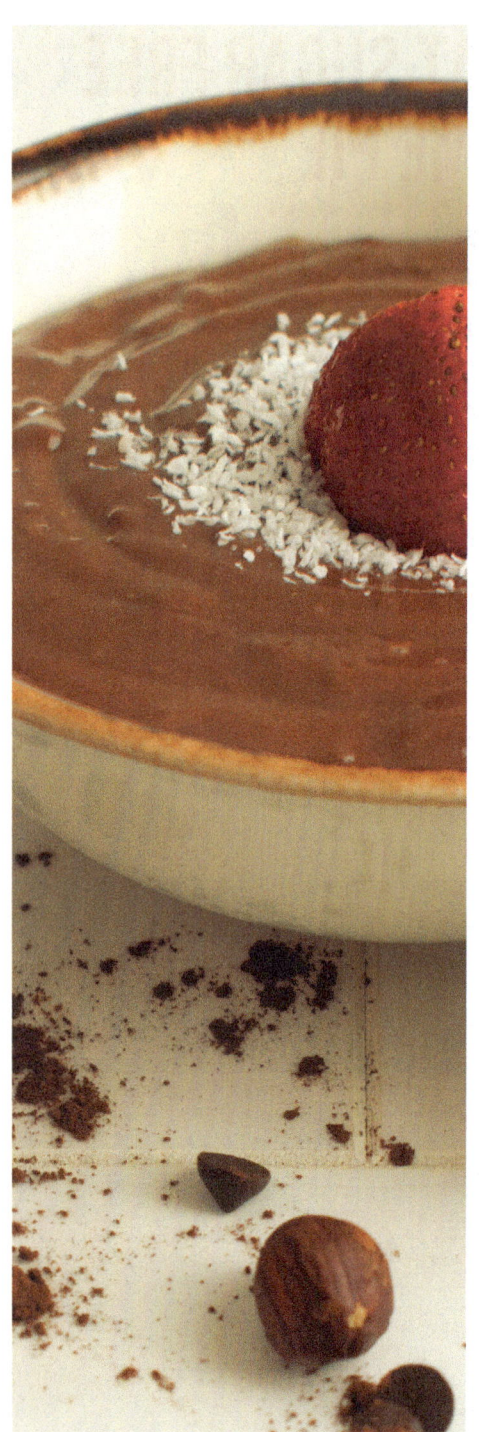

CHOCOLATE PUDDING WITH OLIVE OIL AND SEA SALT

Ingredients:
- 1/2 cup sugar-free chocolate chips
- 1/4 cup olive oil
- 1 teaspoon sea salt

Instructions:
1. In a small saucepan, melt chocolate chips and olive oil over low heat, stirring constantly until smooth.
2. Remove from heat and stir in salt. Pour into individual bowls and let cool completely before serving.

Serving Size: 1/2 cup
Calories: 320

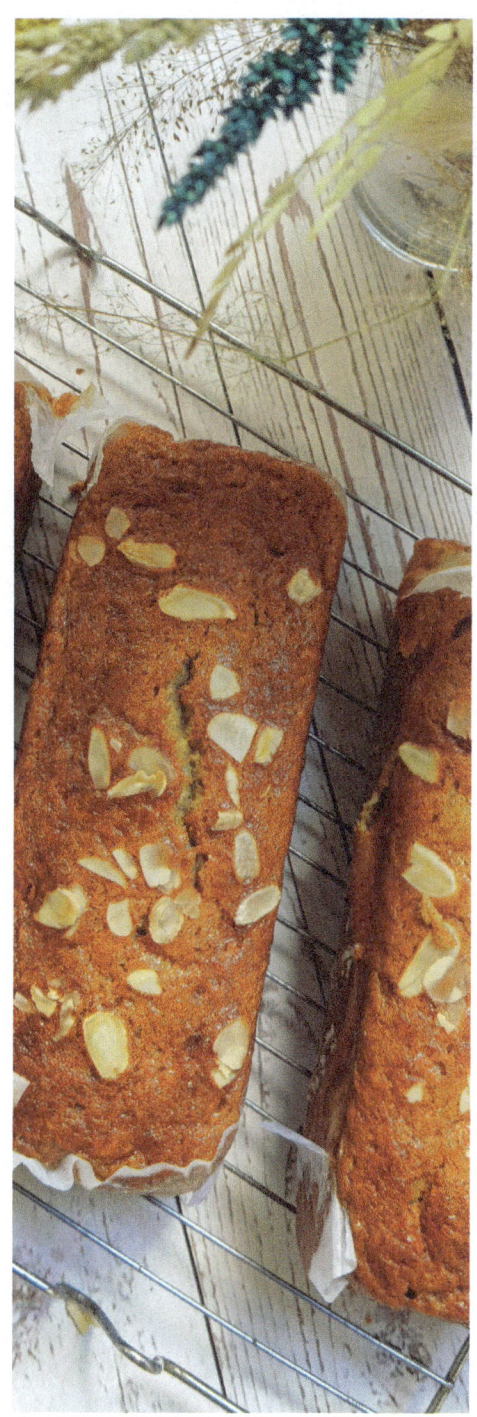

BANANA BREAD

Ingredients:
- 3 ripe bananas, mashed
- 1/3 cup sugar-free syrup
- 1 teaspoon baking soda
- 1 teaspoon vanilla extract
- 1 1/2 cups whole wheat flour blend

Instructions:
1. Preheat oven to 350 degrees F. Grease and flour a 9-inch loaf pan. Set aside.
2. In a large bowl, mix together bananas, sugar-free syrup, baking soda, and vanilla extract. Stir in flour until well combined. Pour into prepared pan.
3. Bake for 45-50 minutes, or until a toothpick inserted in the center comes out clean. Let cool completely before slicing and serving.

Serving Size: 1 slice
Calories: 210

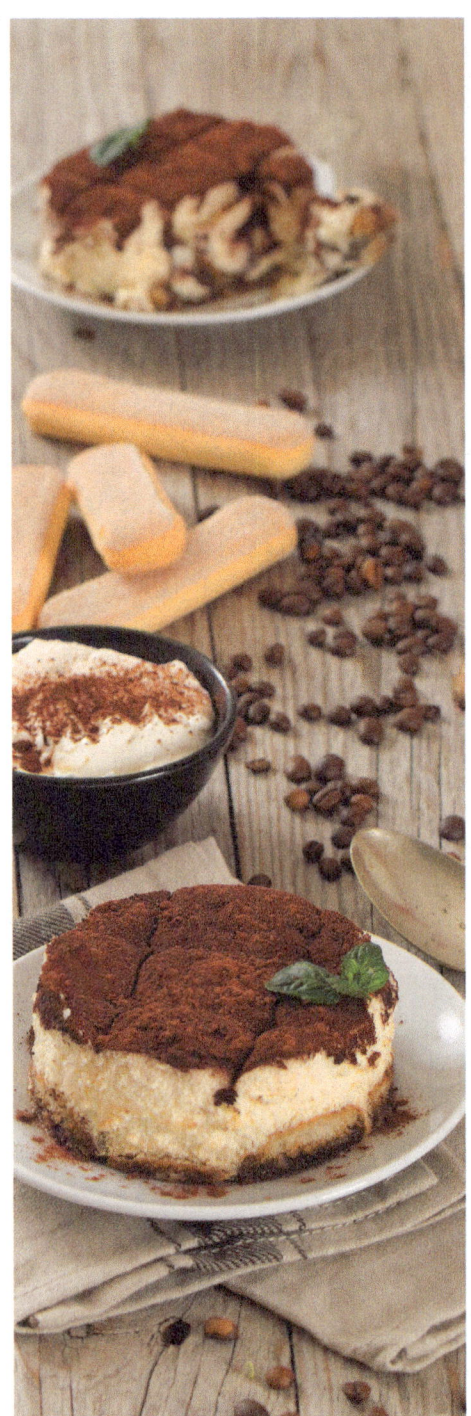

TIRAMISU

Ingredients:
- 1 cup mascarpone cheese
- 1/2 cup heavy cream
- 1/4 cup powdered sugar
- 1 teaspoon vanilla extract
- 24 ladyfingers
- 1/2 cup strong coffee, cooled

Instructions:
1. In a medium bowl, beat together mascarpone cheese, heavy cream, powdered sugar, and vanilla extract until smooth. Set aside.
2. Line the bottom of an 8-inch square pan with half of the ladyfingers. Brush with coffee. Spread with half of the mascarpone mixture. Repeat layers.
3. Cover and refrigerate for at least 2 hours before serving.

Serving Size: 1 piece
Calories: 260

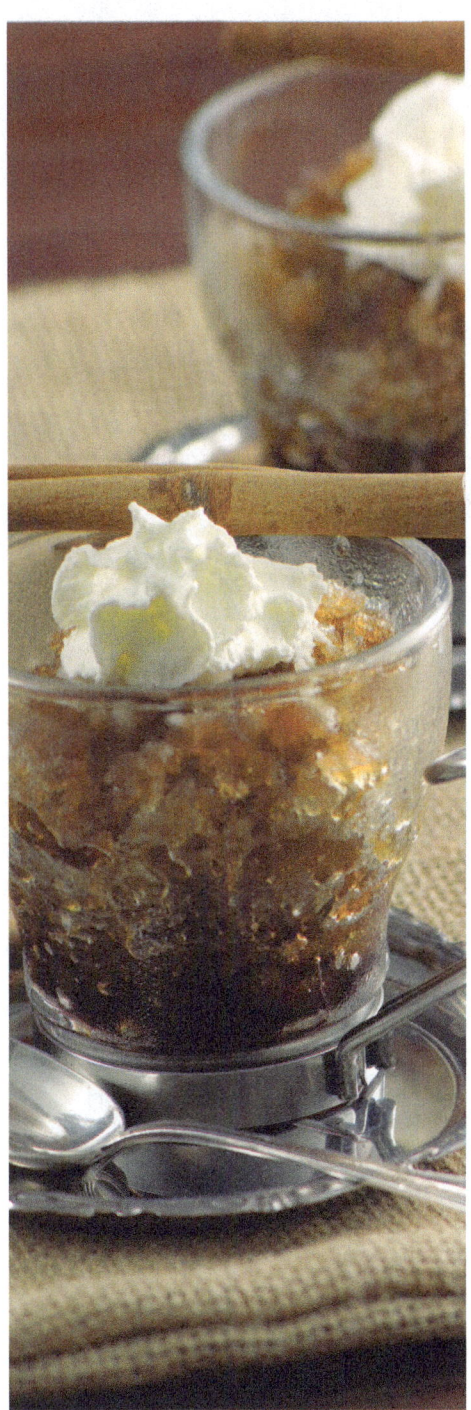

ESPRESSO GRANITA

Ingredients:
- 1 cup water
- 1 cup sugar-free syrup
- 1 tablespoon instant coffee granules

Instructions:
1. In a medium saucepan, bring water and sugar-free syrup to a boil. Remove from heat and stir in coffee granules until dissolved. Pour into a 9-inch square pan.
2. Freeze for 2 hours, or until almost solid. Scrape with a fork to form crystals. Cover and freeze for at least 2 hours before serving.

Serving Size: 1/2 cup
Calories: 100

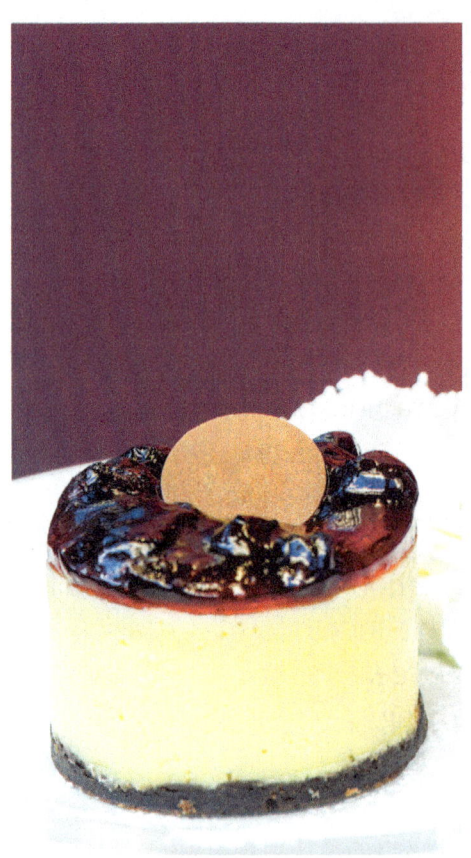

RICOTTA CHEESECAKE WITH WARM BLUEBERRIES

Ingredients:

For the crust:
- 1 1/2 cups graham cracker crumbs
- 3 tablespoons sugar-free syrup
- 6 tablespoons melted butter or margarine

For the filling:
- 2 (15-ounce) containers ricotta cheese
- 1/2 cup sugar-free syrup
- 3 tablespoons all-purpose flour or gluten-free all-purpose flour blend
- 1 teaspoon vanilla extract

Instructions:

1. Preheat oven to 350 degrees F. Grease and flour a 9-inch springform pan. Set aside.
2. In a medium bowl, mix together graham cracker crumbs, sugar-free syrup, and melted butter or margarine. Press into the bottom of the prepared pan. Set aside.
3. In a large bowl, beat together ricotta cheese, sugar-free syrup, flour, and vanilla extract until smooth. Pour into crust.
4. Bake for 60 minutes, or until the center is set. Let cool completely on a wire rack before serving. Serve with warm blueberries, if desired.

Serving Size: 1 piece
Calories: 560

The Complete Anti-Inflammatory Cookbook For Weight Loss   126

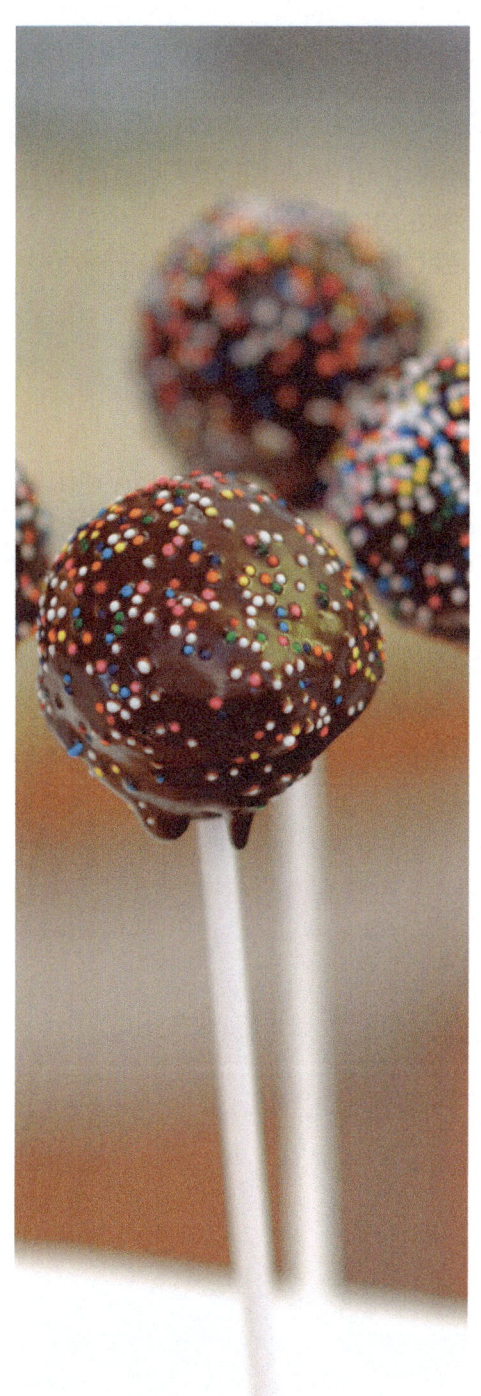

BROWNIE CAKE POPS WITH SPRINKLES

Ingredients:
- 1 (16-ounce) package sugar-free brownie mix
- 1/4 cup water
- 2 tablespoons oil

For the coating:
- 1 (12-ounce) package sugar-free chocolate chips
- 3 tablespoons shortening or coconut oil
- Sprinkles, for decorating

Instructions:

1. Preheat oven to 350 degrees F. Grease and flour a 9x13 inch baking pan. Set aside.
2. In a large bowl, mix together brownie mix, water, and oil until well combined. Pour into prepared pan and spread evenly. Bake for 25 minutes, or until a toothpick inserted in the center comes out clean. Let cool completely before cutting into squares.
3. To make the coating, melt together chocolate chips and shortening or coconut oil in a microwave-safe bowl, stirring every 30 seconds until smooth.
4. Dip the end of a popsicle stick into the melted chocolate and insert into the side of a brownie square. Dip the brownie pop into the melted chocolate, letting any excess drip off. Decorate with sprinkles and place on a wax paper-lined baking sheet. Repeat with remaining brownies. Let chocolate harden before serving.

Serving Size: 1 pop
Calories: 180

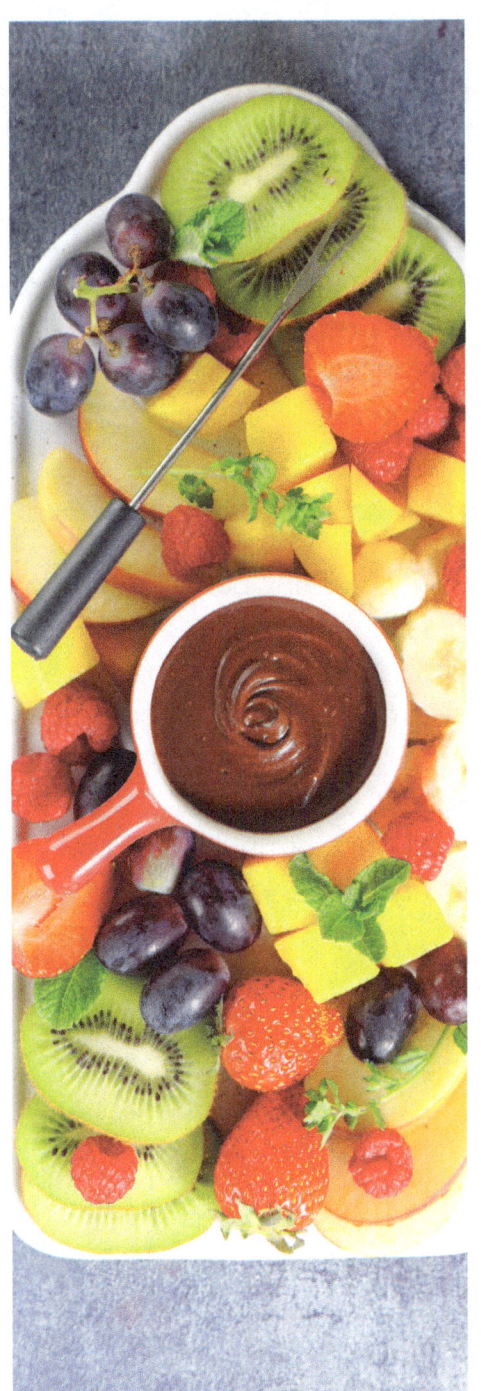

CHOCOLATE-DIPPED FRUIT POPS

Ingredients:
- 1 cup strawberries, halved
- 1 cup blueberries
- 1 cup raspberries
- 1/4 cup sugar-free chocolate chips

Instructions:
1. Thread fruit onto popsicle sticks, alternating between types of fruit. Place in the freezer for at least 2 hours.
2. Melt chocolate chips in a microwave-safe bowl, stirring every 30 seconds until smooth.
3. Dip the frozen fruit pops into the melted chocolate, letting any excess drip off. Place on a wax paper-lined baking sheet and freeze for at least 1 hour before serving.

Serving Size: 1 pop
Calories: 80

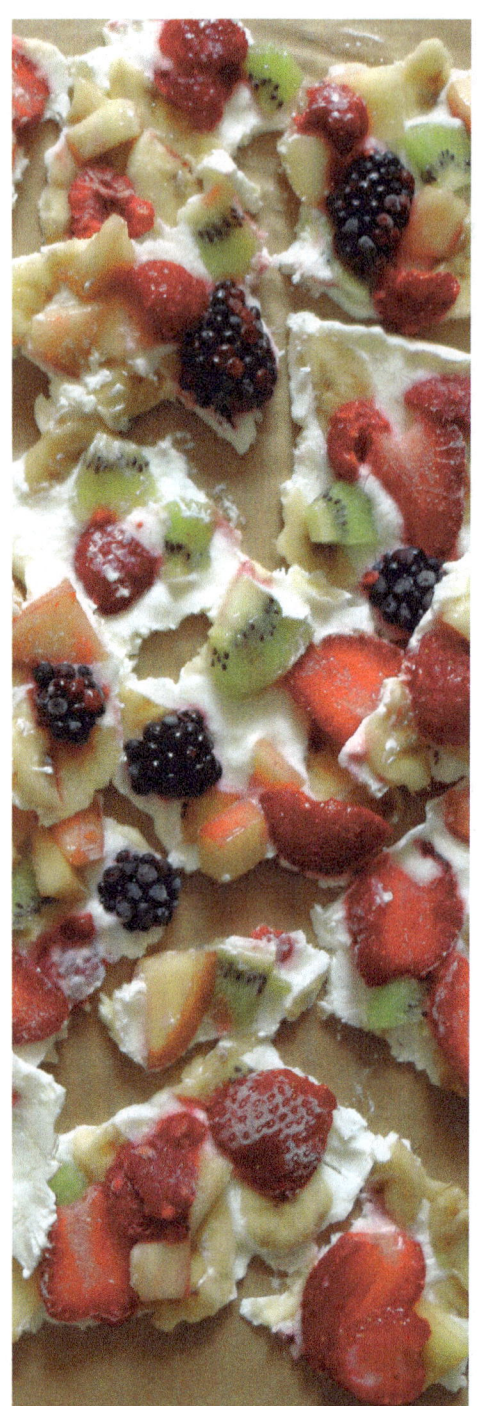

FROZEN YOGURT BARK WITH FRUITS AND NUTS

Ingredients:

- 6 cups vanilla yogurt
- 1 cup strawberries, diced
- 1/2 cup blueberries
- 1/4 cup raspberries
- 1/4 cup chopped nuts

Instructions:

1. Line a 9x13 inch baking pan with wax paper. Set aside.
2. In a large bowl, mix together yogurt, strawberries, blueberries, raspberries, and chopped nuts. Pour into prepared pan and spread evenly.
3. Freeze for 2 hours, or until firm. Break into pieces and serve.

Serving Size: 1 piece
Calories: 150

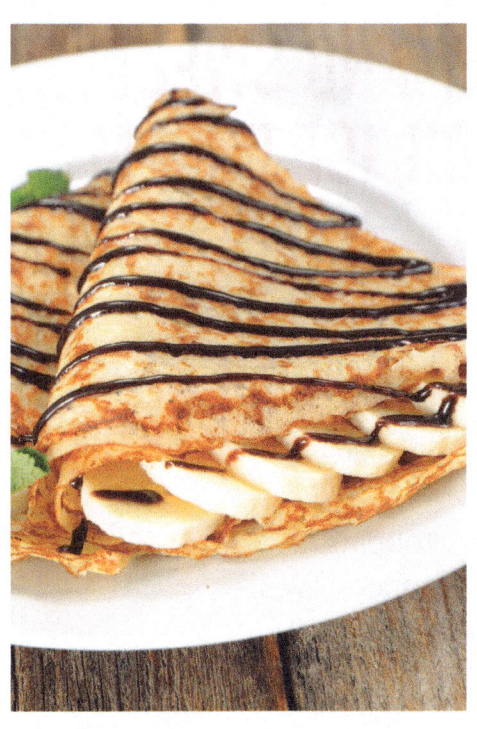

BANANA-NUTELLA CREPES

Ingredients:
- 1 cup all-purpose flour blend
- 2 tablespoons sugar-free syrup
- 1 teaspoon baking powder
- 1/4 teaspoon salt
- 1 1/2 cups milk
- 3 tablespoons melted butter or margarine
- 2 bananas, sliced
- 1/4 cup sugar-free chocolate hazelnut spread

Instructions:
1. In a large bowl, whisk together flour, sugar-free syrup, baking powder, and salt. Slowly add milk, whisking until well combined. Stir in melted butter or margarine.
2. Heat a crepe pan or skillet over medium heat. Grease with cooking spray. Pour 1/4 cup batter into the center of the pan and swirl to spread evenly. Cook for 1-2 minutes, or until the crepe is set and lightly browned. Flip and cook for an additional 1 minute. Repeat with remaining batter.
3. To assemble, place a crepe on a plate and top with banana slices and chocolate hazelnut spread. Roll up and serve immediately.

Serving Size: 2 crepes
Calories: 260

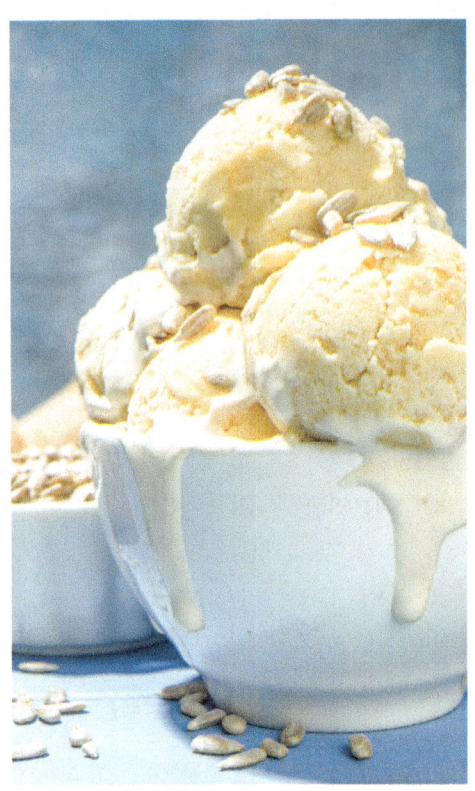

SAVORY AND SWEET OLIVE OIL ICE CREAM

Ingredients:
- 1 cup whole milk
- 1 cup heavy cream
- 1/2 cup sugar-free syrup
- 1 teaspoon vanilla extract
- 1/8 teaspoon salt

For the savory topping:
- 1/4 cup chopped olives
- 1 tablespoon olive oil

For the sweet topping:
- 1/4 cup sugar-free chocolate chips

Instructions:
1. In a large bowl, whisk together milk, heavy cream, sugar-free syrup, vanilla extract, and salt. Pour into an ice cream maker and freeze according to manufacturer's instructions.
2. To make the savory topping, mix together chopped olives and olive oil in a small bowl. Set aside.
3. To make the sweet topping, melt chocolate chips in a microwave-safe bowl, stirring every 30 seconds until smooth. Set aside.
4. To assemble, scoop ice cream into bowls and top with savory or sweet toppings. Serve immediately.

Serving Size: 1/2 cup
Calories: 320

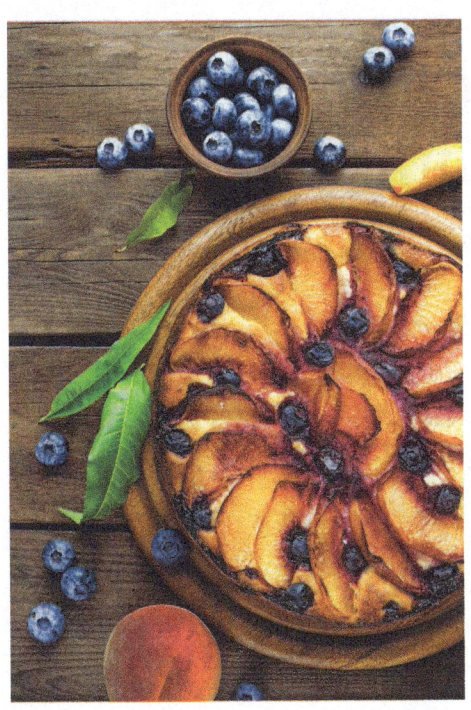

PEACH AND BLUEBERRY GREEK YOGURT CAKE

Ingredients:

- 1 1/2 cups all-purpose flour
- 1 teaspoon baking powder
- 1/4 teaspoon salt
- 3/4 cup Greek yogurt
- 1/2 cup sugar-free syrup
- 1/4 cup olive oil
- 2 eggs, beaten
- 1 teaspoon vanilla extract
- 1 cup peaches, diced
- 1/2 cup blueberries

Instructions:

1. Preheat oven to 350 degrees F. Grease and flour an 8x8 inch baking dish. Set aside.
2. In a large bowl, whisk together flour, baking powder, and salt. In another bowl, mix together yogurt, sugar-free syrup, olive oil, eggs, and vanilla extract. Stir wet ingredients into dry ingredients until well combined. Fold in peaches and blueberries. Pour batter into prepared dish.
3. Bake for 30-35 minutes, or until a toothpick inserted into the center of the cake comes out clean. Allow to cool before serving.

Serving Size: 1 piece
Calories: 380

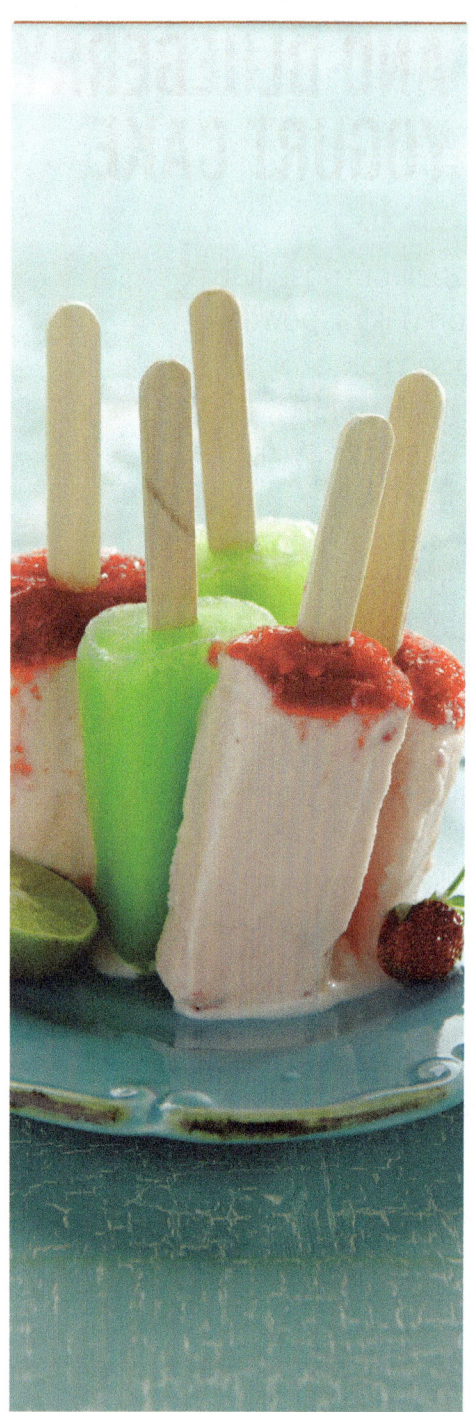

FRUIT-PACKED MEXICAN PALETA

Ingredients:
- 1 cup strawberries, diced
- 1/2 cup raspberries
- 1/2 cup blueberries
- 1 kiwi, peeled and diced
- 1/4 cup sugar-free syrup

Instructions:
1. In a medium bowl, mix together strawberries, raspberries, blueberries, kiwi, and sugar-free syrup.
2. Pour mixture into ice pop molds or small paper cups. Freeze for 2 hours, or until firm. Serve immediately.

Serving Size: 1 paleta or paper cup
Calories: 80

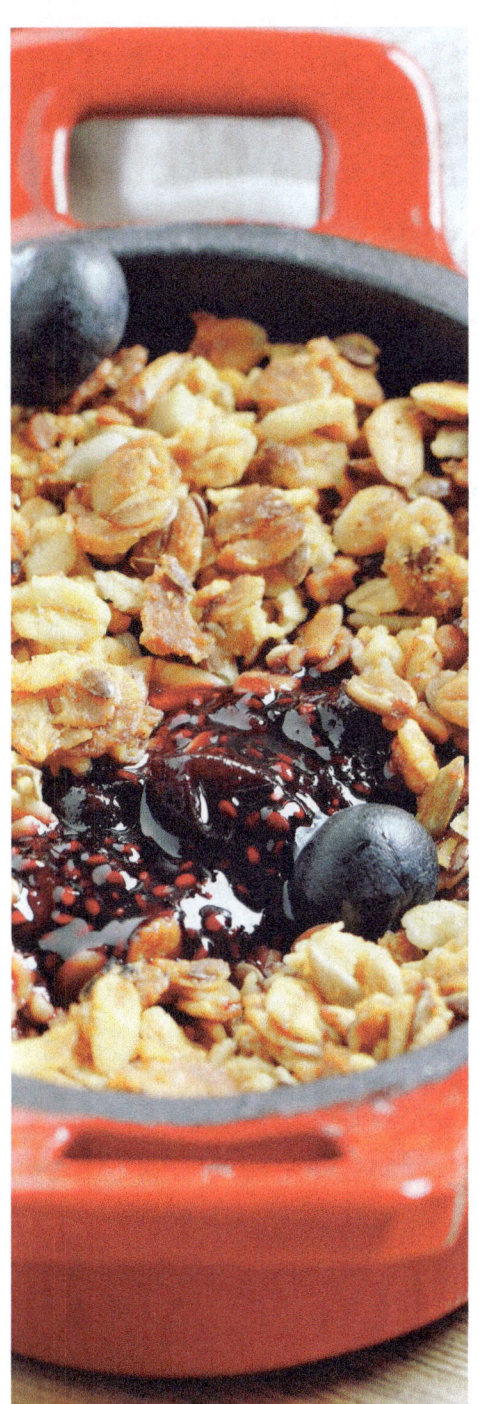

NECTARINE BLUEBERRY CRISP

Ingredients:
- 6 nectarines, diced
- 1 cup blueberries
- 1/2 cup all-purpose flour
- 1/2 cup quick-cooking oats
- 1/4 cup sugar-free syrup
- 1 teaspoon ground cinnamon

Instructions:
1. Preheat oven to 375 degrees F. Grease and flour an 8x8 inch baking dish. Set aside.
2. In a large bowl, mix together nectarines, blueberries, flour, oats, sugar-free syrup, and cinnamon. Pour mixture into prepared dish.
3. Bake for 25-30 minutes, or until the fruit is bubbly and the topping is golden brown. Serve immediately.

Serving Size: 1/2 cup
Calories: 160

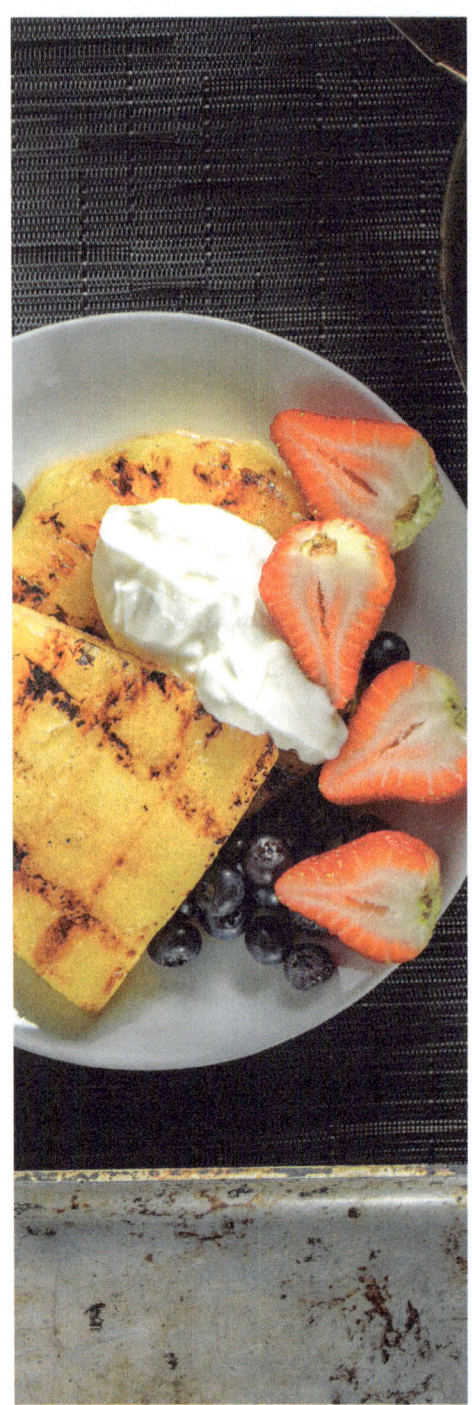

GRILLED PINEAPPLE WITH VANILLA GREEK YOGURT

Ingredients:
- 1 pineapple, sliced into rounds
- 1 cup vanilla Greek yogurt

Instructions:
1. Preheat grill to medium-high heat.
2. Grill pineapple rounds for 2-3 minutes per side, or until grill marks appear and the fruit is slightly softened.
3. Serve grilled pineapple with a dollop of vanilla Greek yogurt.

Serving Size: 1/2 pineapple round + 2 tablespoons yogurt
Calories: 210

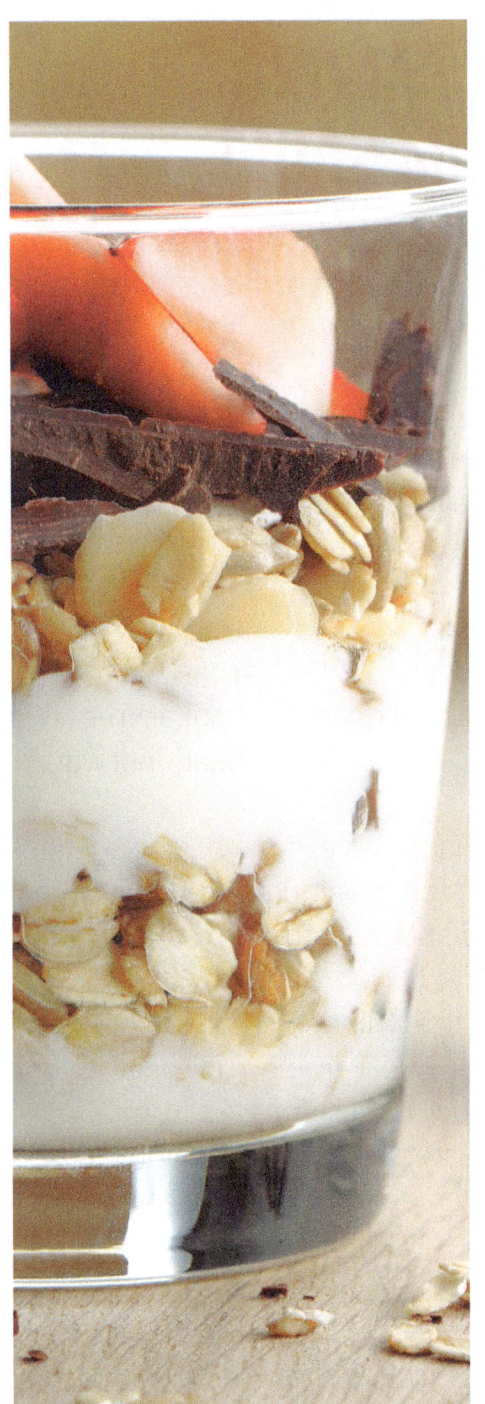

ROASTED STRAWBERRY RHUBARB PARFAITS

Ingredients:
- 4 cups strawberries, diced
- 2 cups rhubarb, diced
- 1/4 cup sugar-free syrup

For the whipped cream:
- 1 cup heavy cream
- 1/4 cup sugar-free syrup

Instructions:
1. Preheat oven to 375 degrees F.
2. In a large bowl, mix together strawberries, rhubarb, and sugar-free syrup. Pour mixture onto a baking sheet and roast for 20-25 minutes, or until the fruit is soft and slightly caramelized. Allow to cool.
3. To make the whipped cream, beat heavy cream and sugar-free syrup together in a large bowl until stiff peaks form.
4. To assemble, layer roasted fruit and whipped cream in glasses or jars. Serve immediately.

Serving Size: 1/2 cup
Calories: 320

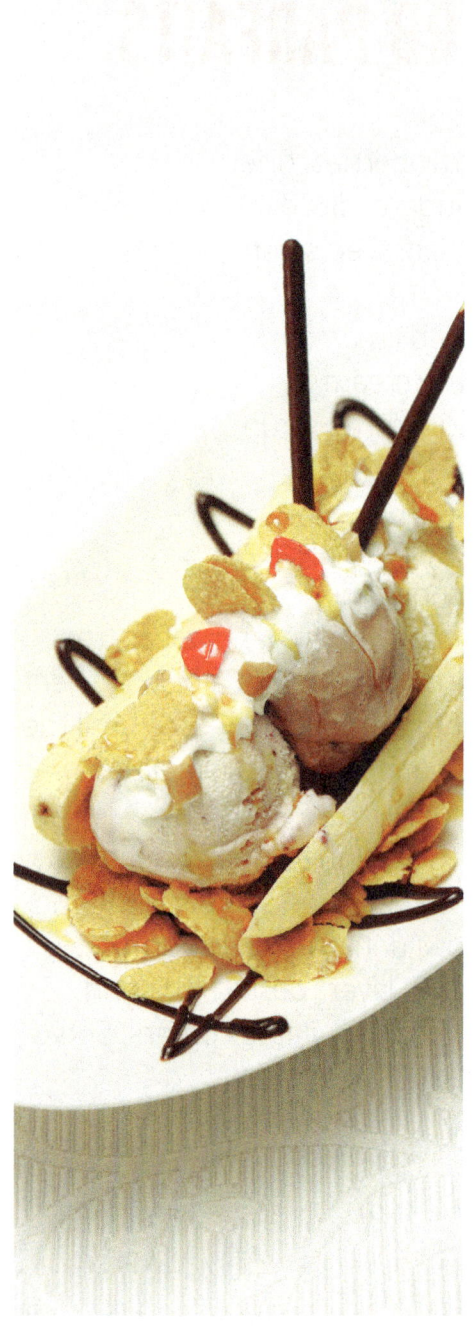

WARM BANANA SPLIT IN A RUM SAUCE

Ingredients:
- 4 bananas, sliced in half lengthwise
- 1 cup sugar-free syrup
- 1/4 cup rum

For the whipped cream:
- 1 cup heavy cream
- 1/4 cup sugar-free syrup

Instructions:
1. Preheat oven to 375 degrees F.
2. In a small saucepan, heat sugar-free syrup and rum over low heat until warm. Set aside.
3. Place banana halves on a baking sheet and roast for 10 minutes. Remove from oven and spoon warm rum sauce over bananas.
4. To make the whipped cream, beat heavy cream and sugar-free syrup together in a large bowl until stiff peaks form.
5. Serve roasted bananas with a dollop of whipped cream and a drizzle of rum sauce.

Serving Size: 1 banana half + 2 tablespoons whipped cream + 1 tablespoon rum sauce
Calories: 260

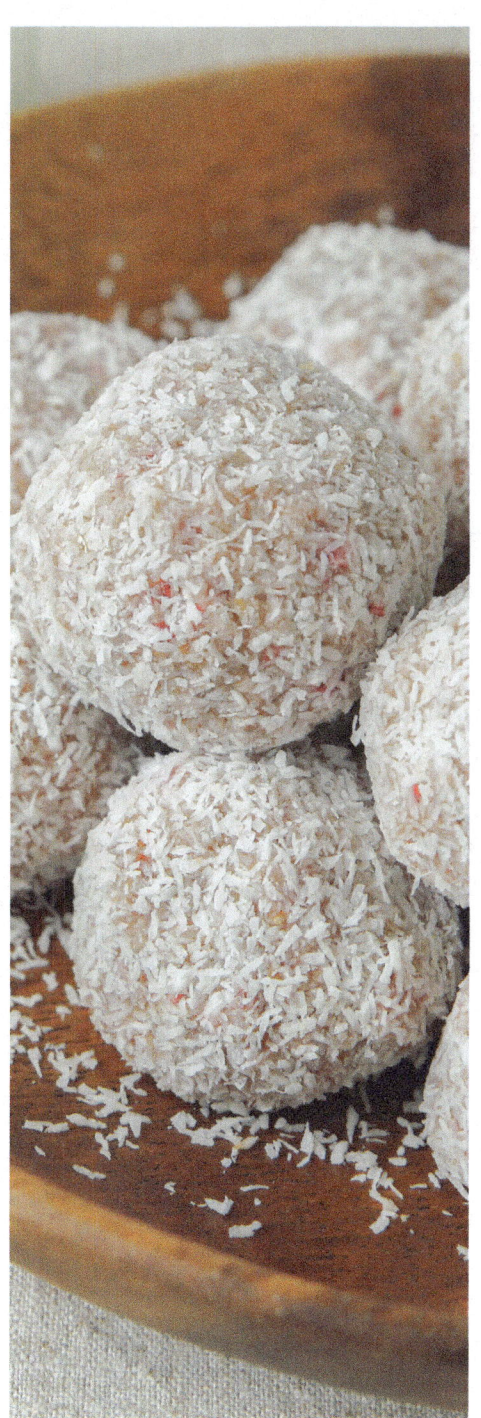

RASPBERRY COCONUT OIL BITES

Ingredients:
- 1 cup raspberries, frozen
- 1/4 cup coconut oil, melted
- 1 tablespoon sugar-free syrup

Instructions:
1. Line a baking sheet with parchment paper and set aside.
2. In a food processor or blender, puree raspberries until smooth. Pour raspberry puree into a small bowl and mix in coconut oil and sugar-free syrup.
3. Place mixture in the freezer for 10 minutes, or until slightly firm. Using a spoon or fork, scoop out raspberry mixture and shape into bite-sized balls. Place on prepared baking sheet and freeze for 1 hour, or until firm. Serve immediately.

Serving Size: 2 raspberry bites
Calories: 70

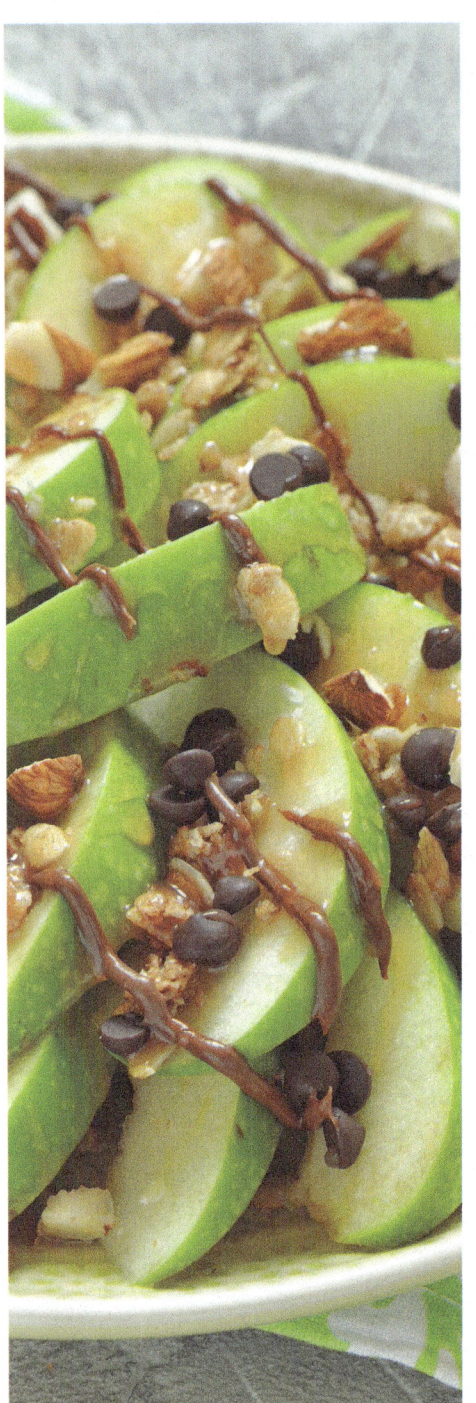

APPLE NACHOS WITH PEANUT BUTTER AND CHOCOLATE SAUCE

Ingredients:
- 2 apples, sliced into thin wedges
- 1/4 cup peanut butter
- 1/4 cup sugar-free chocolate sauce

Instructions:
1. Place apple wedges on a plate or in a bowl.
2. In a small microwave-safe bowl, heat peanut butter and chocolate sauce together for 30 seconds, or until warm. Stir until smooth.
3. Drizzle peanut butter and chocolate sauce over apples and serve immediately.

Serving Size: 1/2 apple + 1 tablespoon peanut butter sauce + 1 tablespoon chocolate sauce
Calories: 190

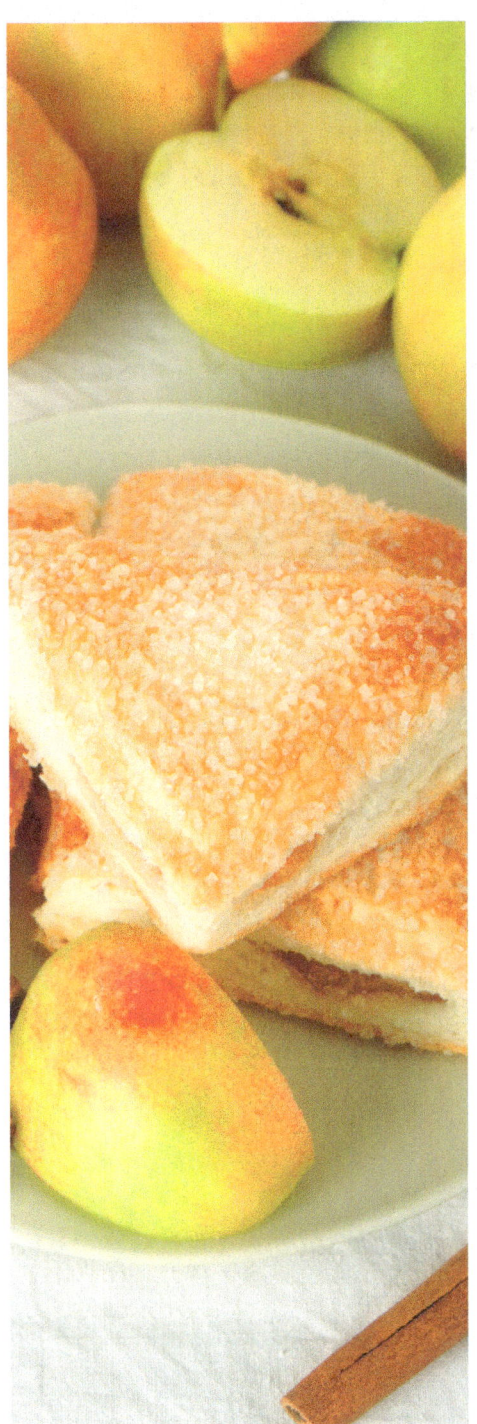

APPLE TURNOVERS

Ingredients:
- 2 apples, peeled and diced
- 1/4 cup sugar-free syrup
- 1 tablespoon sugar-free preserves
- 1 teaspoon ground cinnamon

Instructions:
1. Preheat oven to 375 degrees F.
2. In a small bowl, mix together apples, sugar-free syrup, sugar-free preserves, and ground cinnamon. Set aside.
3. To make the turnovers, cut two 12-inch squares of parchment paper. Place one square of parchment paper on a work surface and spoon apple mixture onto the center of the paper. Top with the second square of parchment paper and crimp the edges together to form a pocket.
4. Place turnover pockets on a baking sheet and bake for 15-20 minutes, or until the apples are soft and the parchment paper is golden brown. Serve warm.

Serving Size: 1 turnover
Calories: 150

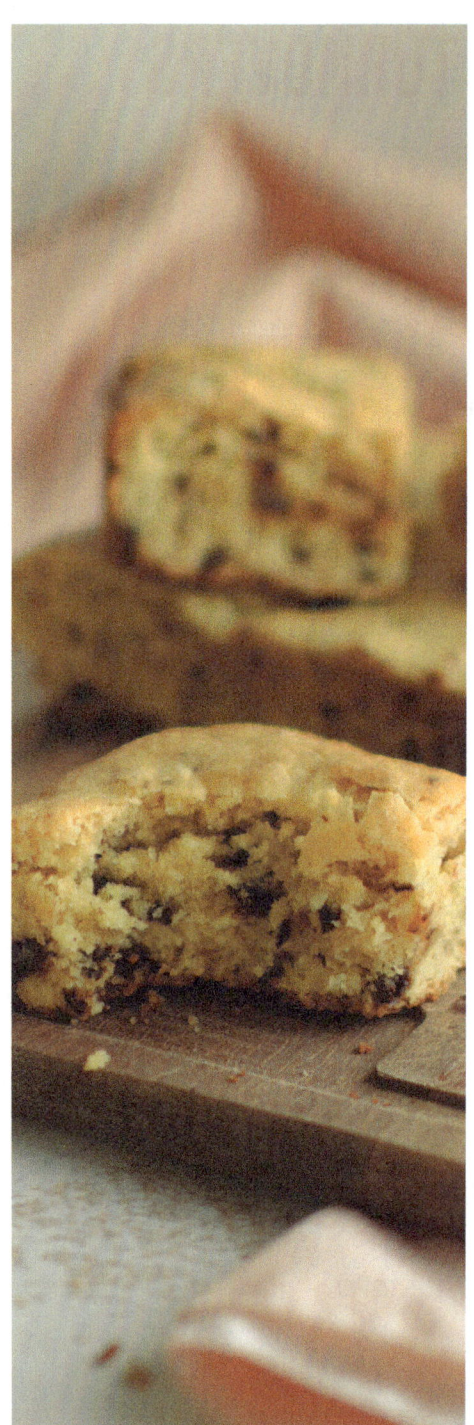

PEANUT BUTTER & CHOCOLATE CHICKPEA BLONDIES

Ingredients:

- 1 can chickpeas, drained and rinsed
- 1/2 cup peanut butter
- 1/4 cup sugar-free chocolate chips
- 1 teaspoon baking powder

Instructions:

1. Preheat oven to 350 degrees F. Line an 8x8 inch baking dish with parchment paper and set aside.
2. In a food processor or blender, combine all ingredients and blend until smooth. Pour mixture into prepared pan and spread evenly.
3. Bake for 20-25 minutes, or until the blondies are firm to the touch. Allow to cool completely before cutting into squares. Serve immediately.

Serving Size: 1 blondie square
Calories: 140

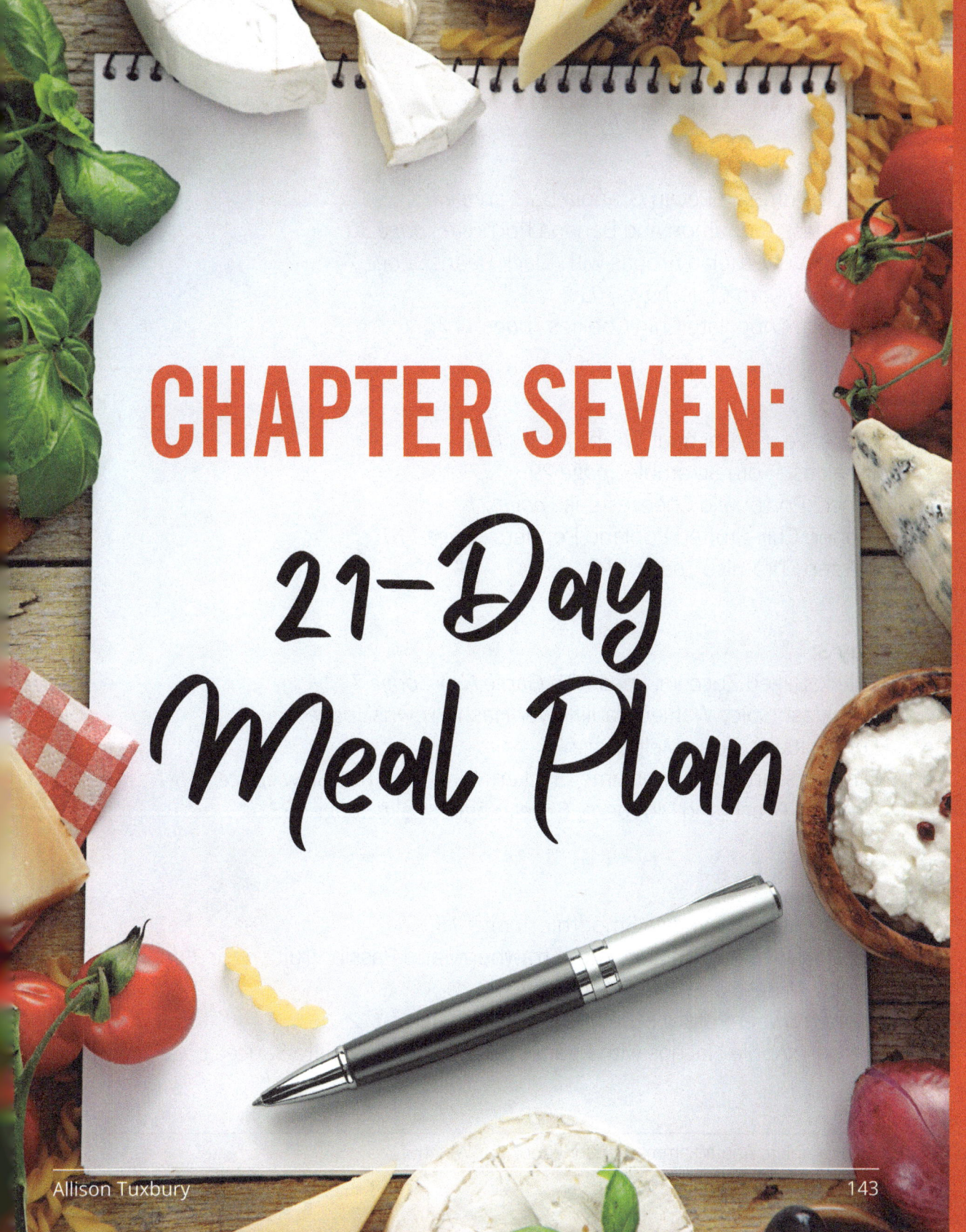

CHAPTER SEVEN:

21-Day Meal Plan

21-DAY MEAL PLAN

Day 1:
Snack: Pumpkin Pecan Granola Bars ..*page 6*
Breakfast: Cinnamon and Banana Porridge ..*page 30*
Lunch: Venezuelan Arepas with Black Beans ..*page 74*
Dinner: Vegan Chili ..*page 103*
Dessert: Chocolate Chip Cookies ..*page 117*

Day 2:
Snack: Veggie Coconut Wraps ..*page 11*
Breakfast: Tofu Scramble ..*page 29*
Lunch: Portobello Cheesesteak ..*page 71*
Dinner: Chili-Stuffed Poblano Peppers ..*page 110*
Dessert: Tiramisu ..*page 124*

Day 3:
Snack: Baked Zucchini Fries with Garlic Aioli ..*page 7*
Breakfast: Spicy Waffled Cauliflower Hash Browns ..*page 36*
Lunch: Italian Tuna Melt ..*page 76*
Dinner: Seared Coconut Lime Chicken With Snap Pea Slaw ..*page 115*
Dessert: Peach and Blueberry Greek Yogurt Cake ..*page 133*

Day 4:
Snack: Fruit and Veggie Smoothie ..*page 15*
Breakfast: Overnight Oats with Strawberry and Passionfruit ..*page 39*
Lunch: Minestrone with Pesto ..*page 78*
Dinner: Sweet Potato & Bean Quesadillas ..*page 112*
Dessert: Apple Nachos with Peanut Butter and Chocolate Sauce ..*page 140*

Day 5:
Snack: Cucumber Avocado Sushi Rolls ..*page 24*
Breakfast: Breakfast Loaded Sweet Potato ..*page 46*
Lunch: Gnocchi with Peas and Prosciutto ..*page 77*
Dinner: Harissa and Citrus Baked Salmon ..*page 102*
Dessert: Peanut Butter & Chocolate Chickpea Blondies ..*page 142*

Day 6:
Snack: Greek Yogurt with Honey and Berries ..*page 25*
Breakfast: Fig, Nut, and Seed Bread with Ricotta and Fruit ..*page 49*
Lunch: Grilled Cheese and Tomato Soup ..*page 72*
Dinner: Chicken Teriyaki Bowls With Cauliflower Rice ..*page 95*
Dessert: Warm Banana Split in a Rum Sauce ..*page 138*

Day 7:
Snack: Oven Baked Cinnamon Apple Chips ..*page 24*
Breakfast: Whole Grain Pancakes With Cashew Butter ..*page 48*
Lunch: Chicken Tortilla Soup ..*page 67*
Dinner: Curried Cod With Coconut Rice ..*page 91*
Dessert: Brownie Cake Pops with Sprinkles ..*page 128*

Day 8:
Snack: Fruit Salad Skewers ..*page 5*
Breakfast: Breakfast Salad with Eggs ..*page 34*
Lunch: Garlic Chili Chickpea Patties ..*page 75*
Dinner: Sheet-Pan Italian Pork Chops ..*page 93*
Dessert: Espresso Granita ..*page 125*

Day 9:
Snack: Avocado Roll-Ups ..*page 2*
Breakfast: Butternut Squash Hash with Fried Eggs ..*page 45*
Lunch: Healthy Crab Cakes with Mango-Avocado Salsa ..*page 81*
Dinner: Chipotle Chicken Fajitas ..*page 86*
Dessert: New York Cheesecake ..*page 119*

Day 10:
Snack: Cucumber Bites ..*page 3*
Breakfast: Quinoa Egg Muffins with Tomato, Basil and Mozzarella ..*page 54*
Lunch: Dilled Salmon with Roasted Asparagus ..*page 83*
Dinner: Carrot Biryani ..*page 90*
Dessert: Lebanese Rice Pudding ..*page 118*

Day 11:
Snack: Cucumber Mint Water ..*page 9*
Breakfast: Smashed Chickpea Bruschetta ..*page 28*
Lunch: Instant Pot Pakistani Chana Dal ..*page 65*
Dinner: Prawn, Fennel, and Asparagus Risotto ..*page 94*
Dessert: Fruit-Packed Mexican Paleta ..*page 134*

Day 12:
Snack: Chocolate Covered Banana Bites ..*page 13*
Breakfast: Mediterranean Breakfast Burrata ..*page 31*
Lunch: Green Frittata ..*page 63*
Dinner: Simple Sesame Chicken with Green Beans ..*page 100*
Dessert: Grilled Pineapple with Vanilla Greek Yogurt ..*page 136*

Day 13:
Snack: Healthy Caramel Pear Dip ..*page 18*
Breakfast: Low-Sugar Cranberry Orange Scones ..*page 33*
Lunch: Artichoke-Feta Quiche ..*page 58*
Dinner: Rich Paprika Seafood Bowl ..*page 104*
Dessert: Apple Turnovers ..*page 141*

Day 14:
Snack:Vegan Energy Balls ..*page 16*
Breakfast: Sweet Potato, Bean, and Kale Shakshuka ..*page 37*
Lunch: Italian Panini with Provolone, Peppers, and Arugula ..*page 56*
Dinner: Summer Fish Stew ..*page 106*
Dessert: Raspberry Coconut Oil Bites ..*page 139*

Day 15:
Snack: Apple Donuts ..*page 20*
Breakfast: Sheet-Pan Vegan Sausage and Vegetables ..*page 42*
Lunch: Caprese Sandwich ..*page 60*
Dinner: Roasted Cauliflower Tacos with Chipotle Cream ..*page 113*
Dessert: Nectarine Blueberry Crisp ..*page 135*

Day 16:
Snack: No-Bake Oatmeal Bars ..*page 4*
Breakfast: Watermelon and Berry Salad with Buckwheat ..*page 47*
Lunch: Mediterranean Chicken Wrap ..*page 64*
Dinner: Broccoli Veggie Pasta Primavera ..*page 114*
Dessert: Frozen Yogurt Bark with Fruits and Nuts ..*page 130*

Day 17:
Snack: Roasted Sweet Potato Wedges with Cinnamon Sugar ..*page 8*
Breakfast: Crunchy Oat Clusters with Peach and Yogurt ..*page 53*
Lunch: Pasta Salad with Lentils, Pesto, and Beans ..*page 73*
Dinner: Spiced Grilled Eggplant with Fresh Tomato Salad ..*page 108*
Dessert: Chocolate Pudding With Olive Oil and Sea Salt ..*page 122*

Day 18:
Snack: Honeydew Melon with Prosciutto ..*page 10*
Breakfast: Curried Chickpea Salad Wraps ..*page 51*
Lunch: Carne Asada Burritos ..*page 79*
Dinner: One Skillet Lemon Chicken and Bell Peppers and Spinach ..*page 107*
Dessert: Low-Fat Sugar-Free Key Lime Pie ..*page 121*

Day 19:
Snack: Vegan Cashew Queso with Broccoli ..*page 12*
Breakfast: Sweet Potato Banana Muffins ..*page 43*
Lunch: Chinese Garlic Tofu Stir Fry ..*page 80*
Dinner: Creamy Chicken Quinoa Broccoli Casserole ..*page 98*
Dessert: Savory and Sweet Olive Oil Ice Cream ..*page 132*

Day 20:
Snack: Homemade Fruit Leather ..*page 17*
Breakfast: Vegan Breakfast Burrito ..*page 32*
Lunch: Chopped Chicken and Broccoli Salad ..*page 62*
Dinner: Seared Tilapia With Spiralized Zucchini ..*page 92*
Dessert: Roasted Strawberry Rhubarb Parfaits ..*page 137*

Day 21:
Snack: Roasted Beet Hummus with Carrot Sticks ..*page 22*
Breakfast: Quinoa Breakfast Bowl with Peanut Butter and Banana ..*page 40*
Lunch: Curried Lentil Soup ..*page 57*
Dinner: Tempeh Lettuce Wraps ..*page 97*
Dessert: Banana-Nutella Crepes ..*page 131*

About The Author

ABOUT ALLISON TUXBURY

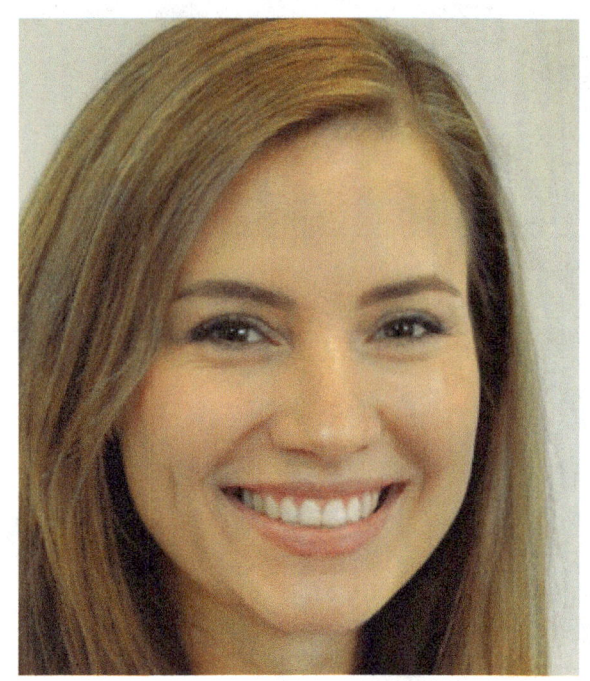

Allison Tuxbury is a professional photographer, digital graphic designer, and lover of food.

She suffered from chronic health conditions and autoimmune symptoms for nearly two decades before finding solutions in meditation, alternative medicines, energy therapy, breathwork, and nutritional meals that fuel the body.

She writes because she loves to share what she's learned with the world, and because it's fun to come up with new meals.

She hopes that through her books others who also suffer from ailments will find relief and recovery as well. She currently lives in Texas with her three children and husband.

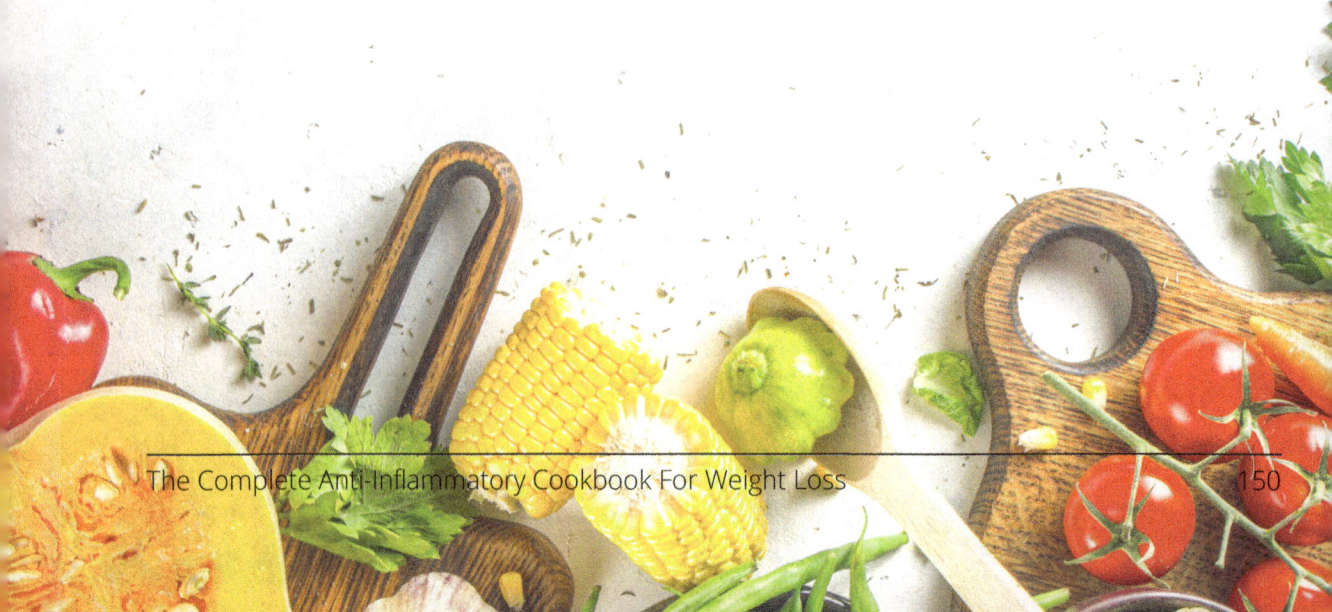

INDEX

A
- Apple Donuts..20
- Apple Nachos with Peanut Butter and Chocolate Sauce..140
- Apple Turnovers..141
- Artichoke-Feta Quiche..58
- Asian Chicken Lettuce Wraps..70
- Avocado Roll-Ups..2
- Avocado Soup..105
- Avocado Toast with Egg..35

B
- Baked Zucchini Fries with Garlic Aioli..7
- Banana Bread..123
- Banana-Nutella Crepes..131
- Blueberry Pie..120
- Breakfast Loaded Sweet Potato..46
- Breakfast Salad with Eggs..34
- Broccoli Veggie Pasta Primavera..114
- Brownie Cake Pops with Sprinkles..128
- Butternut Squash Hash with Fried Eggs..45

C
- Caprese Sandwich..60
- Carne Asada Burritos..79
- Carrot Biryani..90
- Chargrilled Lamb and Veggie Sandwich..68
- Chia Seed Pudding with Almond Milk and Fresh Fruit..26
- Chicken Pot Stickers..61
- Chicken Teriyaki Bowls With Cauliflower Rice..95
- Chicken Tortilla Soup..67

- Chickpea Scramble with Tomato and Avocado..41
- Chili-Stuffed Poblano Peppers..110
- Chinese Garlic Tofu Stir Fry..80
- Chipotle Chicken Fajitas..86
- Chocolate Chip Cookies..117
- Chocolate Covered Banana Bites..13
- Chocolate Pudding With Olive Oil and Sea Salt..122
- Chocolate-Dipped Fruit Pops..129
- Chopped Chicken and Broccoli Salad..62
- Cinnamon and Banana Porridge..30
- Creamy Chicken Quinoa Broccoli Casserole..98
- Crunchy Oat Clusters with Peach and Yogurt..53
- Cucumber Avocado Sushi Rolls..24
- Cucumber Bites..3
- Cucumber Mint Water..9
- Curried Chickpea Salad Wraps..51
- Curried Cod With Coconut Rice..91
- Curried Lentil Soup..57

D
- Dilled Salmon with Roasted Asparagus..83

E
- Espresso Granita..125

F
- Fig, Nut, and Seed Bread with Ricotta and Fruit..49
- Frozen Yogurt Bark with Fruits and Nuts..130

INDEX

- Fruit and Veggie Smoothie..15
- Fruit Salad Skewers..5
- Fruit-Packed Mexican Paleta..134

G
- Garlic Chili Chickpea Patties..75
- Gnocchi with Peas and Prosciutto..77
- Greek Yogurt with Honey and Berries..25
- Green Frittata..63
- Grilled Cheese and Tomato Soup..72
- Grilled Pineapple with Vanilla Greek Yogurt..136

H
- Harissa and Citrus Baked Salmon..102
- Healthy Caramel Pear Dip..18
- Healthy Crab Cakes with Mango-Avocado Salsa..81
- Homemade Fruit Leather..17
- Honeydew Melon with Prosciutto..10

I
- Instant Pot Pakistani Chana Dal..65
- Italian Panini with Provolone, Peppers, and Arugula..56
- Italian Tuna Melt..76

L
- Lebanese Rice Pudding..118
- Low-Fat Sugar-Free Key Lime Pie..121
- Low-Sugar Cranberry Orange Scones..33

M
- Mediterranean Breakfast Burrata..31
- Mediterranean Chicken Wrap..64
- Minestrone with Pesto..78
- Miso-Roasted Eggplant Steaks with Sweet Potatoes..85
- Moo Shu Mushroom Wraps..109
- Mushroom Crostini With Herbs And Garlic..22

N
- Nectarine Blueberry Crisp..135
- New York Cheesecake..119
- No-Bake Oatmeal Bars..4

O
- One Skillet Lemon Chicken and Bell Peppers and Spinach..107
- Oven Baked Cinnamon Apple Chips..24
- Overnight Oats with Strawberry and Passionfruit..39

P
- Parmesan Zucchini Chips..21
- Pasta Salad with Lentils, Pesto, and Beans..73
- Peach and Blueberry Greek Yogurt Cake..133
- Peanut Butter & Chocolate Chickpea Blondies..142
- Portobello Cheesesteak..71
- Prawn, Fennel, and Asparagus Risotto..94
- Pumpkin Pecan Granola Bars..6

INDEX

Q
- Quinoa Breakfast Bowl with Peanut Butter and Banana..40
- Quinoa Egg Muffins with Tomato, Basil and Mozzarella..54

R
- Raspberry Coconut Oil Bites..139
- Rich Paprika Seafood Bowl..104
- Ricotta Cheesecake with Warm Blueberries..126
- Roasted Beet Hummus with Carrot Sticks..22
- Roasted Cauliflower Tacos with Chipotle Cream..113
- Roasted Chicken and Potato With Kale Salad..88
- Roasted Strawberry Rhubarb Parfaits..137
- Roasted Sweet Potato Wedges with Cinnamon Sugar..8

S
- Savory and Sweet Olive Oil Ice Cream..132
- Seared Coconut Lime Chicken With Snap Pea Slaw..115
- Seared Tilapia With Spiralized Zucchini..92
- Sheet-Pan Italian Pork Chops..93
- Sheet-Pan Vegan Sausage and Vegetables..42
- Simple Sesame Chicken with Green Beans..100
- Smashed Chickpea Bruschetta..28
- Spiced Grilled Eggplant with Fresh Tomato Salad..108

- Spicy Avocado Toasted Muffin with Shaved Ham and Spinach..52
- Spicy Waffled Cauliflower Hash Browns..36
- Stuffed Dates with Almond Butter..14
- Summer Fish Stew..106
- Sweet Potato & Bean Quesadillas..112
- Sweet Potato Banana Muffins..43
- Sweet Potato, Bean, and Kale Shakshuka..37

T
- Tempeh Lettuce Wraps..97
- Tiramisu..124
- Tofu Scramble..29

V
- Vanilla and Cinnamon Breakfast Rice..38
- Vegan Breakfast Burrito..32
- Vegan Cashew Queso with Broccoli..12
- Vegan Chili..103
- Vegan Energy Balls..16
- Vegan Spinach and Sun-Dried Tomato Pasta..69
- Veggie Coconut Wraps..11
- Venezuelan Arepas with Black Beans..74

W
- Warm Banana Split in a Rum Sauce..138
- Watermelon and Berry Salad with Buckwheat..47
- Whole Grain Pancakes With Cashew Butter..48

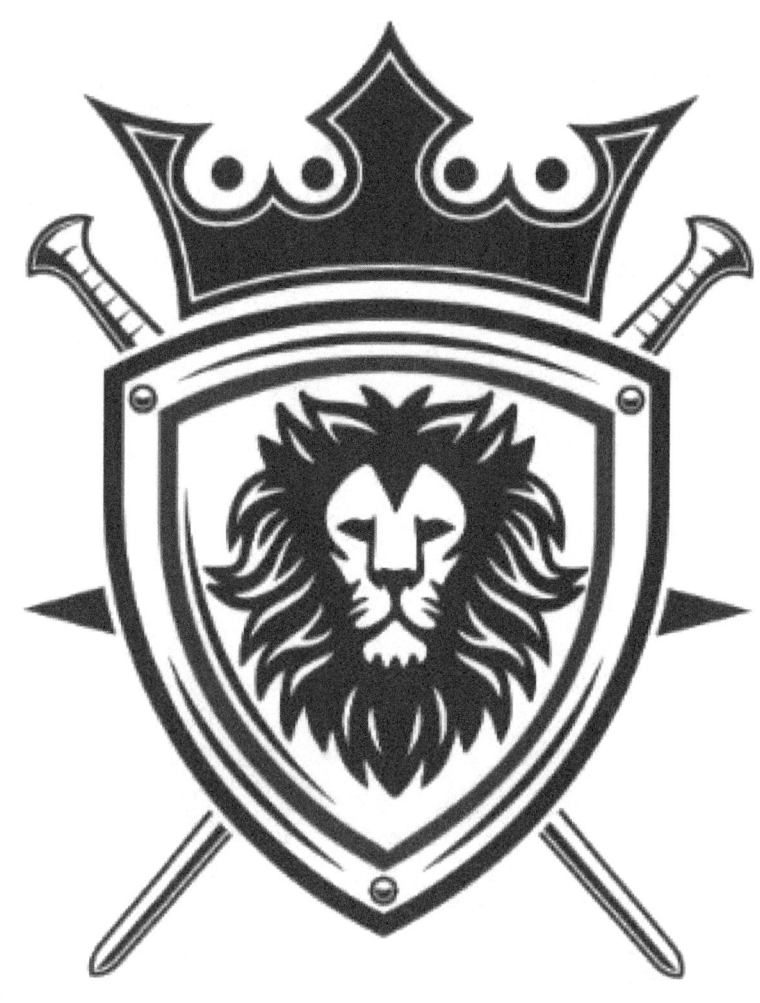

Made in the USA
Coppell, TX
11 June 2023

17945226R00098